Effects of High Altitude on Human Birth

Observations on Mothers, Placentas, and the Newborn
in Two Peruvian Populations

Effects of High Altitude
on Human Birth

Observations on Mothers, Placentas,
and the Newborn in Two Peruvian
Populations

Jean McClung

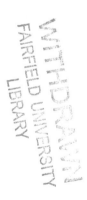
Harvard University Press

Cambridge, Massachusetts

1969

To Bob Dylan

Foreword

At several places around the globe man and domestic animals live at altitudes higher than 4,000 meters. Prominent among these locations are the Andean Highlands of Peru, Bolivia, Chile, and Argentina, where some 12,000,000 people live, and the Himalayan Highlands, where live a comparable number.

The nature and sequence of human adaptations to high altitude have fascinated physiologists for decades. Studies at high altitude stations in Peru, Colorado, and Switzerland have revealed changes in cardiovascular physiology in man, sheep, and other animals living at these altitudes. Increases in red cell mass, hematocrit, and viscosity of blood have been demonstrated, as well as hyperventilation and pulmonary hypertension. More recent studies by L. A. Sobrevilla and others in Peru have revealed changes in endocrine functions that occur regularly at high altitudes.

The observation that human beings and domestic animals adapted to low altitudes may experience reproductive difficulties when they move to high altitudes is an ancient one, dating back at least to the settlement of Peru by the Spaniards in the sixteenth century. In this book, Jean McClung examines the question in detail and shows that it is not simply an old wives' tale but a real phenomenon. She goes further, to ask whether the Indians who have lived in their highlands for two millennia or more have undergone genetic adaptations that enable them to reproduce under such conditions. Do the members of tribes that have lived for generations at high altitude have a physiological advantage over their lowland cousins in their ability to reproduce?

McClung's carefully controlled studies of births in hospitals in Lima and Cuzco show that the weight of the placenta is not reduced in births at high altitude, even though the birth weights of the Cuzco infants are, on the average, more than 200 grams less than those of the Lima infants. The area of the Cuzco placentas was greater than those in Lima, even though the weights were the same, for they had a greater diameter and lesser depth than those from deliveries in Lima.

The differences in birth weight do not appear to result from racial differences, for Cuzco-born women who move to Lima give birth to infants that weigh as much as the infants of Lima-born mothers. Furthermore, the birth weights of babies born in Cuzco of European mothers are below the average birth weight of the lowland population. Careful anthropometric measurements of mothers and neonates have shown no difference in the nutritional status of the two populations. The lower birth weight at high altitude is not the result of premature delivery of the child nor of maternal or fetal malnutrition; apparently the major contributing factor is fetal hypoxia. Even in sea-level pregnancies the oxygen tension in fetal blood and tissues is less than that in maternal blood. These findings have led Sir Joseph Barcroft to remark that the usual hypoxia of the fetus resembles "Everest in utero." When the mother herself is on Everest, or halfway up Everest, the increased fetal hypoxia puts these fetuses at a substantial extra risk, which is reflected in decreased birth weight and increased fetal and neonatal mortality. The increased placental area in the highland pregnancies reported in this book may represent an adaptation designed to increase gas exchange and minimize hypoxia. The physiological and chemical factors that regulate the size and shape of the placenta under these conditions constitute another fascinating problem for future investigation.

CLAUDE A. VILLEE

Preface

This study of human adaptation to high altitude began in the spring of 1966. I had become interested in the subject at Radcliffe, while writing a paper on the Aymara Indians of Bolivia for a course in the physical anthropology of living races. Dr. Albert Damon, instructor in the course, suggested I write to Professor Paul Baker of the Pennsylvania State University, who was heading a long-range investigation of the physical anthropology of high altitude populations in the southern Peruvian highlands. With the encouragement of Dr. Baker, I applied for and was granted a traveling fellowship from the Harvard Committee on Latin American Studies for study in Peru during the summer of 1966.

The specific project plan was conceived during a discussion with Dr. Baker, who mentioned that Dr. Emilio Picon-Reategui, a Peruvian biochemist who had worked at the Pennsylvania State University laboratory in Nuñoa, Peru, was interested in placental and birth weights at high altitude. Peruvian physicians had reported smaller than average newborns with very large placentas in highland hospitals. A test of these observations was not feasible in the small rural population in the Nuñoa sample, but might be possible in Cuzco, a nearby provincial capital with a modern hospital. In a hospital setting at the Cuzco altitude of 11,200 feet, I could examine mother, newborn, and placenta in eighty or more births, which would be a statistically meaningful sample. Using identical methods, I could then study a sample of births in a Peruvian hospital at sea level among a racially and socially similar population. With these relatively controlled observations I hoped to verify and quantify previous reports that the high altitude environment significantly alters human pregnancy and birth.

Dr. Damon and Dr. Baker have been of continuing help in this project, as have many others. Members of the Pennsylvania State research team contributed time, equipment, and advice. In particular, Brooke Thomas supplied valuable background on previous investigations in Peru and on its climate, economy, and culture; A. Roberto Frisancho provided the Quechua translation of the fertility questionnaire; and in Nuñoa, Richard and Jeanne Mazess offered helpful criticism during my first analysis of the data from Cuzco. Dr. Shirley Driscoll, pathologist at the Boston Lying-In Hospital, spent many afternoons instructing me in laboratory techniques of placental pathology, orienting me in the medical literature, and interpreting the results of the study.

My work in Cuzco would not have been possible without the assistance of Dr. Romulo Acurio, pediatrician at the Hospital Regional. Dr. Horacio Chavez of the Division of Obstetrics was also of help in arranging laboratory space and training the staff to assist me. Dr. Abelardo Temoche of the Peruvian Department of Public Health made possible my entrance into the Lima hospital, the Maternidad de Lima, where Dr. Jose Pereda, hospital pathologist, provided kind and patient assistance. The entire staff of both hospitals—from aides and janitors to nurses, midwives, doctors, and hospital administrators—did a remarkable job of adapting to the novel requirements of the study. Staff members rescued placentas from disposal heaps, recorded anthropometric measurements, corrected my Quechua, and waylaid departing mothers so that I could interview them. They also provided me with meals, lodging, and companionship. My gratitude extends, as their help extended, far beyond the limits of the project. The mothers included in the study sample were also extraordinarily helpful, translating for me to the Quechua-speakers in the ward, correcting my mistakes, and forcing me to explain frequently and simply what I was doing and why it was important.

The project design and analysis of results have been aided by reprints, correspondence, and unpublished data from many scientists working on altitude or the placenta. Chief among these are Drs. J. S. Stickney and Edward Van Liere of the University of West Virginia; Dr. Kurt Benirschke of Dartmouth Medical School; Dr. James Metcalfe of the University of Oregon Medical School; Dr. Richard Naeye of the University of Vermont College of Medicine; Dr. Orlando Alzamora of Chulec Hospital in La Oroya, Peru; Dr. Toshio Fujikara of the National Institutes of Health; Dr. Irwin Kaiser of the University of Utah Medical Center; and Drs. Giles Toll and Lula Lubchenco of Denver, Colorado. The Library of the San Marcos Facultad de Medicina in Lima made special provision for me to read unpublished papers and to copy materials, as did the West Virginia Medical Library.

The staff of the Harvard Computation Center helped greatly in punching, sorting, printing, and programing the data. Henry Harpending of the Harvard Department of Anthropology did the initial error analysis of the anthropometry, and Mary Hyde of the Department of Social Relations gave needed advice on format and analysis of results of the Data-Text program. Others at Harvard who encouraged me were Drs. William Howells and Douglas Oliver of the Department of Physical Anthropology and Dr. Claude Villee of the Harvard Medical School.

The placental examination form presented in Appendix I was sent to Dr. Stanley Garn of the International Biological Program for use in preparing a standard form for placental examination in societies under study in the Program. Anthropometric data from this study will be used by A. Roberto Frisancho in a comparative study of growth in Quechua populations living in various environments. A summary of this work was delivered at the 1967 Meetings of the American Association of Physical Anthropologists, and some of its data on placental pathology and birth weight was presented by Dr. James Metcalfe at a 1968 conference on cardiovascular disorders in pregnancy.

Contents

Tables

xv

Figures

Chapter I Theoretical Considerations

The major stimulus for the study of human birth at high altitude has come from clinical observations and clinical problems. Physicians have reported that at high altitude newborn babies are generally small in size and the rates of prematurity and neonatal mortality are high.

Additional stimulus comes from the biological sciences. Animal studies indicate that pregnancy at high altitudes places severe stress on both the altitude tolerance and reproductive capacity of the mother. Many of the maternal variables such as heart size, blood volume, and body weight, which have been correlated with fetal development and birth weight in sea level populations, are severely affected by acute exposure of the mother to high altitude hypoxia. The mammalian fetus, even at sea level, lives in what might be compared to the oxygen environment of an adult at high altitude. The multiple stresses of high altitude gestation thus offer a natural opportunity for the study of hypoxia, birth, and their interrelationship.

The major tool for the study of human birth at high altitude is also a clinical one—controlled observation and analysis. However, the perspective of biological theory and experiment is important at this stage as well. Many of the multiple factors affecting a variable such as birth weight vary with altitude, and these must be recognized and controlled. Animal experiments identify specific physiological mechanisms leading to observed effects on fertility or fetal develop-

1

ment, which may ultimately be tested in epidemiologic studies of human populations. The significance of differences observed in human high-altitude populations can be confirmed and clarified by comparison with results of animal experiments. For example, observations of high rates of fetal and neonatal mortality among inbred laboratory animals exposed to various experimentally-produced low-oxygen pressures constitute convincing evidence that similar observations made on natural high-altitude populations are due to a real effect of oxygen lack.

In this chapter are described the experiments, observations, and theories that form the biological background for studies of human birth at high altitude. The material is reviewed first with regard to altitude physiology in the adult organism and the effects of hypoxia on the reproductive cycle at all points from gamete formation to gestation. High altitude gestation is then re-examined with respect to its effect on the fetal organism—specifically on fetal growth, survival, and birth weight.

FERTILITY

Carlos Monge, in a series of papers in the 1940's, introduced to science the idea that low oxygen pressure at altitudes of 10,000 feet and over has a detrimental effect on human and animal fertility. His conclusions were based largely on historical, veterinary, and medical impressions. Chronicles of the Spanish conquest record that no child of Spanish blood was born during the first fifty years of Spanish occupation of the Peruvian highlands. According to Monge, the birth rate of Spaniards began to approach that of Andean natives only after the Europeans had inhabited altitudes of 10,000 feet or more for over a generation and had begun to interbreed with the native population. In 1639 the Spaniards moved their capital from the mountains to the seacoast because "horses, fowl and pigs do not produce offspring (Monge, 1948). Monge reported low rates of lambing in high altitude sheep. Imported breeding stock showed temporary and sometimes permanent sterility in the Peruvian Andes, with histological evidence of degeneration of the seminiferous tubules in acclimatizing males. Physicians had the impression that spontaneous abortion and premature labor were more common at high altitudes, and non-native women were usually advised to go to sea level during pregnancy.

Experimental Difficulties and Theoretical Controversies. Monge's speculations are still being tested by animal experiments, but evidence is conflicting. The natural high-altitude environment involves several kinds of physiologic stress; lowered oxygen pressure, cold, low humidity, and high levels of cosmic radiation. Animal experiments on "altitude effects" usually duplicate altitude hypoxia by using pressure chambers, but this procedure introduces handling stress and also neglects interactions between hypoxia and other components of the natural high-altitude environment.

Experiments using natural altitude encounter problems of differentiating acute from long-term altitude effects, and responses of native animals from those of sojourners. Classical physiology asserted that complete acclimatization to oxygen pressures at altitudes of over 10,000 feet is not possible for non-natives. Paul Bert wrote in 1878: "The organisms at present existing on the surface of the earth are acclimated to the degree of oxygen tension in which they live; any decrease, any increase seems to be harmful to them when they are in a state of health" (Hurtado, 1962). Studies of human acclimatization offer an alternative to this hypothesis. Differences observed in individuals transported to high altitude can be interpreted as pathologic changes resulting from hypoxic stress, but they can also be interpreted as adaptive changes leading to a new equilibrium state at the lower oxygen pressure.

An animal introduced to a low oxygen environment typically responds by increasing heart and respiration rates. Hyperventilation reduces blood carbon dioxide and leads to alkalosis. Oxygen-deprived tissues produce an erythropoietic factor that increases production of red blood cells. This "secondary" polycythemia increases blood volume and viscosity, which, with reflex constriction of pulmonary vessels in response to lower oxygen pressure in inspired air, causes pulmonary hypertension and leads to increased heart volume and hypertrophy of the right ventricle. This is the typical response to a low oxygen environment, but there are other mechanisms, in addition to an increase in the oxygen-carrying capacity of the blood, that act to maintain a constant level of respiration at the cellular level. These include an increase in the number of capillaries per unit area, an increase in the size of the red blood cells, and possibly modifications of membranes to facilitate diffusion of oxygen out of the red blood cells and into the tissues. The increases in muscle myoglobin and total Cytochrome C reported in animals exposed to hypoxia are not yet fully understood, but probably reflect modifications in cellular utilization of oxygen (Barbashova, 1964).

Red blood cell count is the standard method of assessing altitude response, but in individual cases it shows poor correlation with functional measures of adaptation, such as ability to do work. Since oxygen is a fundamental requirement for cell metabolism and survival, it is not surprising that animals have many mechanisms for buffering oxygen deprivation, and that the pattern of combination of primary responses varies not only among individuals but in the same individual at different times.

It is possible that some of the intra-individual variation in hypoxia response reflects variations in the individual's adaptation to temperature. It has long been known from laboratory experiments that cold-exposed animals can recover from acute exposures to hypoxia that are several times the lethal level for littermates who have been kept at warm temperatures (Miller and Miller, 1966). The ability of an animal to maintain normal body temperature in a cooled environment under varying atmospheric pressures is used as a laboratory assay of the minimal oxygen pressure a species can tolerate (Folk, 1966). Recent observations on natural populations (Roberts et al., 1966) indicate that deer mice living at altitudes of 10,000 feet have very low metabolic rates in the summer; in the winter their metabolic rates are quite high. Increased metabolic rate is a typical response to cold in these animals, while depression of metabolic rate is a typical mammalian response to chronic hypoxia. These experiments indicate that the quality of an organism's altitude adaptation may vary seasonally. The experiments are, of course, not directly applicable to the human case, but they suggest that cold as well as hypoxia may contribute to the physiological variation found in men at high altitudes. Tests of temperature regulation in Quechua Indians native to high altitude indicate that the natives' response to chronic cold exposure may differ from that of acclimatized whites. Although both groups maintained the same basal metabolic rates during cold exposure, the Indians maintained skin temperature at a higher level, and this heat loss led finally to a decline in rectal temperature (Baker et al., 1967). Monge (1966) has suggested that the short limbs and massive trunk of the Andean Indian are advantageous in resisting cold as well as hypoxic stress.

Alberto Hurtado describes the physiology of native high-altitude man as parallel to that seen in acclimatizing sojourners: high level of erythropoietic activity, slight hypocapnia, large heart and blood volumes, pulmonary hypertension with high residual lung capacity and dilatation of pulmonary capillaries. Natives have slow heartbeats and low peripheral blood pressures that show subnormal increases during exercise. Field studies in progress (Baker et al., 1965) aim to test

Hurtado's observations and relate them to basal metabolism, biochemistry, and changes observed in acute altitude adaptation.

Proponents of Bert's theory of altitude pathology contend that the Andean man must represent a physiologically distinctive human strain (Monge, 1948). Archeology gives evidence of continuous habitation of the southern Peruvian highlands for at least 2,000 years. Human artifacts 10,000 years old have been found in the Andes (Monge and Monge, 1966). Depending on the stringency of altitude as a selective pressure—a point still under debate—this may have been long enough for the population to become genetically specialized. Today twelve million people live at altitudes of 10,000 feet and over in the South American Andes. The only other high-altitude human populations of comparable size are found in the Himalayas. Available reports indicate that the human population above 10,000 feet in the Himalayas is not as dense as that found in the Andes, and the maximum permanently-inhabited altitude is 15,000 feet, in contrast to the 17,500-foot limit in the Andes. Comparatively small and isolated populations at 10,000 feet and over are also found in Ethiopia, parts of the Swiss Alps, and the Rocky Mountains of North America.

The Andean native is short in stature, with little subcutaneous fat and a large thoracic circumference. Monge contends that this is an ideal anatomic framework for maximizing oxygen uptake and minimizing oxygen waste. However, studies at sea level report that thoracic circumference correlates only 0.3–0.4 with vital capacity, while the correlation between stature and vital capacity is 0.6–0.7. (Damon, 1966). Other altitude physiologists contend that the large thoracic circumference is a pathologic rather than an adaptive response to hypoxia (Tenney and Remmers, 1966) and parallels the chest expansion seen in patients with a chronic lung disease, such as emphysema.

Monge uses analogy with other animals native to high altitude as further evidence that the altitude adaptation of Andean man is irreversible and has a genetic basis. The llama, for example, even after generations at sea level exhibits persistence of adaptation to hypoxia—close packing of hemoglobin in red blood cells, longer erythrocyte survival time, and a high affinity of hemoglobin for oxygen (Kreuzer, 1966). Some genetic strains of mice are naturally resistant to the stress of hypoxia (Feigen and Johnson, 1962). Rodents native to high altitudes have high hematocrits that persist through many generations if the animals are brought to sea level. The apparently genetically determined hematocrits of several strains of deer mice vary directly with the altitude of the strain's native habitat (Folk, 1966).

Spanish chronicles attributed the failure of Negro slavery in Peru to the inability of the slaves to acclimatize to high altitudes. Monge theorizes that Negroes are least resistant to hypoxia, Caucasians intermediate, and Mongoloids most adaptable. Worldwide racial distribution at high altitudes tends to support the theory, as do sea level studies that show pulmonary function to be less efficient in Negroes than in whites (Damon, 1966). Most direct observations compare native Indians to Caucasian scientists or to Mestizos. Acute altitude responses of Negroes and the physiology of residents of Negro colonies at high altitude, such as those found in Ecuador, have not been studied.

Studies of respiratory physiology indicate, however, that the altitude adaptation of the Andean Indian is reversible and not qualitatively distinctive from the pattern seen in acclimatizing Europeans. "Acclimatized" natives, as well as sojourners, can "deacclimatize" in a potentially fatal syndrome that resembles polycythemia vera; in "chronic mountain sickness" or "Monge's disease" hyperventilation is replaced by hypoventilation, and the secondary polycythemia normally associated with the altitude response becomes uncontrolled and leads to serious hematologic and neurologic complications (Monge and Monge, 1966).

When Andean natives migrate to low altitudes, erythrocyte level and heart volume decrease to sea level values. Even the large thoracic circumference characteristic of these people seems to be a secondary response to hypoxia rather than a genetic adaptation. Microscopic examination of the lungs of high altitude natives shows congestion of the blood capillaries and sinusoids with dilatation of lung alveoli and thickening of the alveolar walls (Campos R. and Iglesias, 1956). Both microscopic and macroscopic changes in the lungs and thorax are only extreme cases of the changes seen in acclimatizing outsiders. Hurtado (1955) attributes the native advantage at altitude to continuous exposure beginning in intrauterine life and to the cultural necessity for exercise. Outsiders most closely approximate the native adaptation if they reside continuously at high altitude for more than six months and are physically active (Keys, 1936). Hurtado concludes that Andean natives show the same individual variability in respiratory response as non-natives, but are collectively at the adapted end of the continuum of individual adaptive potentials.

Carlos Monge (1948), however, suggests that the decisive adaptation of the Andean race is in reproductive, not respiratory, physiology. It is the fertility advantage of Andean natives at high altitude that makes them racially distinctive.

Evidence for Hypoxia Effects. The fertility-depressing effects of altitude are attributed to secondary responses, tissue changes produced despite adjustments of the circulatory system to maintain oxygenation. Inhibition of fecundity may take place at any step in the reproductive cycle: germ cell production, copulation, fertilization, implantation, gestation, and birth. Reproductive efficiency of a population also depends on the proportion of liveborns surviving to reproductive age.

The hypothalamic and endocrine systems, which control the reproductive cycle, as well as the sex organs themselves, may be affected by high altitude. The high oxygen requirement of the brain places the critical limit on the animal's tolerance to hypoxia, but there is disagreement as to specific functional effects, and maximum tolerance levels are variable (Opitz, 1950). Most recent endocrinologic evidence indicates that rats born and attaining maturity at 3,800 meters of natural altitude have reduced pituitary weight but retain normal adrenal weight (Timiras and Woolley, 1966). This and other studies of endocrine function at high altitude point to a shift of pituitary activity to ACTH (adrenocorticotrophic hormone) production with reduced secretion of the other pituitary trophic hormones. Several studies have shown increased excretion of adrenal steroids in men undergoing acute exposure to high altitudes (Moncloa et al., 1965). The effect is not observed when subjects reacclimatize to low altitudes, so it seems to be a direct effect of hypoxia rather than an artifact resulting from the stress associated with transport. It has been conjectured that the low carbon dioxide levels secondary to hypoxia produce this increase in adrenal activity. Reduction of thyroid activity reported at high altitude may be related to a decreased pituitary secretion of TSH (thyroid stimulating hormone); lowered levels of thyroid hormone would lead to a diminished oxygen requirement and to decreased catabolism of cortisol, both of which seem advantageous under hypoxic conditions (Debias, 1966). Depression of thyroid hormone probably occurs only after chronic exposure to hypoxia; in man the acute response to high altitude is a slight increase in circulating thyroid hormone as reflected by a transitory increase in basal metabolism and a decrease in blood cholesterol (Moncloa et al., 1966). In the Himalayas thyroid deficiency is related to iodine deficiency in the food and water supply (Harrison, 1966), but in the Peruvian Andes iodine deficiency and endemic goiter are uncommon at altitudes of 3,000 meters and over (WHO,

1960). Animal studies show that the effect of hypoxia on the thyroid persists even when iodine intake is adequate.

Growth retardation reported in Andean natives as compared with United States and sea-level Peruvian populations may be associated with a high altitude effect on the pituitary; changes in pituitary activity would be a simple explanation for the effects of hypoxia on fertility that Monge outlined. Baker, using height, weight, and radiographic measures of 78 males and 68 females ranging from one to 25 years of age and living at altitudes of between 13,000 and 17,000 feet in Peru, reports that sexual dimorphism does not appear in them until about the age of 16 years. No data exist on age at menarche in this population, but it probably is not earlier than the first appearance of sex differences in height and weight. Despite an early average age for cohabitation in the population, Baker has observed no births to women under the age of 18. Studies in human populations at lower altitudes support this proposed association between altitude and late maturation. J. A. Valsik (1965), after reviewing several studies of mountain populations in eastern Europe, has estimated that median age at menarche increases by three months for every 100 meters of altitude. The estimate is from uncontrolled data and reflects economic and racial differences associated with altitude as well as a possible physiological effect. Valsik's formula would predict a delay of ten years in age at menarche for girls living at the Andean altitudes of 4,000 meters.

There is little evidence, however, that pituitary function is responsible for these effects. L. A. Sobrevilla and collaborators (1967) measured urinary gonadotrophins in eight sea-level men brought to 14,000 feet for two weeks and in ten men native to that altitude. In this small sample they found no significant difference in urinary gonadotrophins or testicular function. The investigators point out that their methods would not have detected small differences. However, animal experiments have shown that the testicular degeneration which occurs after prolonged exposure to high altitude cannot be prevented by administration of gonadotrophins (Altland and Highman, 1968). It is now possible to measure STH (growth hormone) in the blood directly, using radio-immunoassay. This would be a direct test of one possible relationship of the pituitary to altitude adaptation.

Carl Moore and Dorothy Price (1948) tested growth and reproductive functions of homogeneous laboratory rats reared at 600 feet, 7,500 feet, 9,600 feet, and 14,260 feet of natural altitude. They reported normal growth and maturation in all animals and no effect of altitude on body weights or weights of the endocrine and reproductive organs. Animals at the highest altitude showed 100 percent breeding efficiency. Moore and Price attributed earlier reports of epithelial degeneration in the seminiferous tubules and decreased number and motility of mature spermatozoa to the artificial conditions of pressure chamber experiments.

However, Monge's original observations (1945) on fertility impairment in rats, cats, rabbits, and sheep were made at 4,540 meters (14,800 feet) of natural altitude. More recent animal experiments indicate the six month period used by Moore and Price was not long enough. P. D. Altland (1949) found that fertility impairment first became evident in rats after one year of exposure and increased with time. Most recent experiments indicate that increased altitude, increased time of exposure, and increased physical exertion at high altitude add to the likelihood of histologic changes in the testes. Due to the length of the spermatogenic cycle and the astronomical number of spermatazoa produced, extensive histologic changes in the testes may be unaccompanied by decreased breeding efficiency at high altitude. S. F. Cook and A. A. Krum (1955) reported no fertility effect until the sixth generation of mice born at the 12,500-foot White Mountain Research Station. Average litter size dropped steadily until the twelfth generation, when complete functional sterility was observed in the high altitude mice. It seems unlikely that high altitude was the only factor affecting fertility in this population, but a fire at the research station terminated the experiment before final observations could be made.

W. H. Weihe (1962) reported that the anestrous phase of the menstrual cycle was prolonged in 50 percent of female rats taken to 3,450 meters (11,300 feet) of natural altitude, but this may have been an acute effect due to transport. Other studies report unaltered estrous cycles in rats exposed to simulated altitude (Nelson and Burrill, 1944). The ovaries and uterus have shown little change under experimental anoxia in contrast to the obvious degeneration seen in male reproductive organs (Monge, 1945; Van Liere and Stickney, 1961).

Monge has suggested that altitude also depresses libido and copulation frequency. Rams brought to Morococha (14,-800 feet) did not copulate during the first forty-seven days at this altitude. Psychological effects of acute exposure to hypoxia have been studied by R.A. McFarland (1939). Under hypoxia human subjects showed severe fatigue symptoms. Other investigators have described feelings of lassitude, disorientation, euphoria, or irritability in men exposed to high altitude conditions (Mosso, 1898; Schaffer, 1962). It is not known if Andean altitudes produce psychological effects on long-term residents or what relation the symptoms observed by McFarland would have to copulation frequency. Hurtado (1960) has suggested that primary central nervous system disorder may be responsible for the physiological changes leading to Chronic Mountain Sickness. Monge and Monge (1967) report that the prevalance of epilepsy in Peru seems markedly high. There is evidence that psychoneurological factors can affect even the more automatic steps in the reproductive cycle—ovulation, conception, frequency of spontaneous abortion and of premature birth (Richardson and

Guttmacher, 1967). This is an intriguing area for specula-
tion, but there is little basic understanding of central nervous
system involvement either in hypoxia or in the reproductive
process.

Because of the general cultural uniformity imposed on this
region by the Inca empire, it can be assumed that voluntary
determinants of fertility are similar at all altitudes (Price,
1965). The existing differences, if they have any overall
effect, would seem to favor higher fertility at higher altitudes
where age at cohabitation is lower and trial marriage is
practised. However, the seasonal migration of men in many
high altitude populations to lowland areas for several months
of agricultural work may be a differential involuntary factor
in the high altitude culture that adversely affects fertility
levels (Davis and Blake, 1957). Monge (1948) asserts that
the Incas tried to curb such migration and enforced mass
marriages in the highland areas as part of an effort to maintain high birth rates at high altitudes.

A recent analysis by J. M. Stycos (1968) of Peruvian census
data reveals unexpected influences of altitude and Spanish
culture on fecundity. Using data from the 1940 census, Stycos
calculated the child-woman ratio for each Peruvian province,
that is, the number of children under age six per 100 women
age 20 to 59. He found a highly significant negative correlation (-0.39; $P < 0.1$) between child-woman ratio and altitude of the provincial capital. This would tend to confirm
Monge's hypothesis that fertility is reduced at high altitude.
However, when Stycos considered only those provinces where
more than 50 percent of the population speaks Spanish, the
correlation was reduced and was not significant. Stycos pro-
poses that Spanish culture tends to increase fecundity. When
Spanish marriage customs replace Quechuan permissiveness
about sex, age at cohabitation decreases and the stability of
the cohabiting relationship increases. This increased fecundity
is most prominent in Spanish rural areas; fecundity of both

Spanish- and Indian-speakers is decreased in urban centers. The 1940 data used by Stycos is probably not an accurate census of the Indian community. However, his study indicates the importance of social factors in determining fecundity and the difficulty of isolating purely biological effects of high altitude.

Biological factors affecting fertilization, implantation, and the early stages of gestation are still largely unknown. Animal experiments indicate that the embryo is most sensitive to environmental trauma of all kinds in the period between fertilization and implantation. Resistance of the ovum to sperm penetration, rate of cleavage of the pre-blastula embryo, time of passage through the oviducts, uterine secretions, and endometrial development—all might be sensitive to high altitude hypoxia (Wolstenholme, 1965). Altland (1949) found significantly fewer implantations in breeding female rats exposed seven hours daily to 18,000 feet of simulated altitude: 7.0 implantations per mother at this altitude as compared to 9.0 in sea level controls. Altland also reports that 55.1 percent of implanted fetuses were resorbed at high altitude, as compared to 26.9 percent resorption in sea level controls.

It is important to remember that the high altitude environment includes aspects other than hypoxia which may affect fertility. Maternal nutrition, for example, is determined by the types of edible plants and animals available in the ecological system specific to any altitude. Barley grain and potato tubers, staples of the human diet at high altitudes in Peru, contain large amounts of plant estrogens (Hafez, 1967). If consumed in adequate quantities, these plant estrogens could lead to hyperplasia of the uterine endometrium, aberrations in the estrous cycle, and decreased fertility. There is no evidence that plant estrogens are in fact a significant determinant of reproductive pathology in the Andes.

In summary, available evidence tends to support Monge's

contention that high altitude depresses fertility. Animal experiments have shown that hypoxia has detrimental effects on sperm formation and on the early stages of gestation. Such effects would be expected on the basis of other neurological and endocrinological effects of hypoxia. Conflicting results in experiments testing these fertility effects may be due to differences in the type and degree of hypoxic stress, in duration of exposure, in the amount of confounding physiological stress—particularly cold stress—and in the species used in the experiment. If high altitude does have severe detrimental effects on fertility, genetic as well as physiological adaptations to hypoxia may be necessary for the survival of a population at high altitude.

PREGNANCY

Most studies of altitude effects on gestation have focused on the later stages of pregnancy, which are easier to study—stillbirth frequency, birth weight, and infant viability. These stages are important in respect to the possible selective pressure exerted by hypoxia on high altitude populations. Increased death rates in the late fetal and neonatal periods form a more effective check on population increase than either increased abortion rate or moderately decreased fertility. The later in the life of the conceptus that death occurs, the longer the mother is prevented by gestation and later inhibited by lactational amenorrhea from conceiving another and perhaps viable fetus (Perrin and Sheps, 1965). Furthermore, A. H. Smith and U. K. Abbott's work with domestic birds (1961) indicates that these later stages mark a critical phase in the reproductive cycle at high altitude. White Leghorns taken to the White Mountain Research Station at 12,500 feet showed normal laying patterns, and egg fertility was 93 percent of the sea level value. However, hatchability—the percent of fertilized eggs hatching—was only 3 percent of the normal value, and hatching time was prolonged 15 percent.

Eggs laid at 12,500 feet and taken to sea level for hatching showed 75 percent of normal hatchability but retained the longer high-altitude hatching time. After six generations at high altitude the Leghorns had increased hatchability to 30 percent of normal, and hatching time was normal.

In mammals exposed to high altitude the situation is more complex and provides an excellent system in which to study interactions among endocrinologic, circulatory, and genetic mechanisms of altitude adaptations. Altitude effects reach the fetus via the composition of the nutrient maternal blood, as modified by the placenta. The fetus, which has an independent circulatory system, can respond to hypoxia with primary mechanisms—such as high hematocrit and the high affinity of fetal hemoglobin for oxygen—as well as with secondary mechanisms relating to tissue uptake of oxygen. Mother, placenta, and fetus are secreting hormones during gestation that may be affected by hypoxia and may modify oxygen consumption and uptake. The mother's thyroids and adrenals double in weight during pregnancy; fetal pituitary, thyroid, and adrenal are active in the human fetus by the fifth month of gestation (Anderson, 1966), and placental growth hormones are probably important regulators of fetal size (Dancis, 1965; Ounsted, 1966).

Postulated racial and strain differences in altitude tolerance could also be tested in this system. Portions of the placenta, the decidua capsularis and the decidua basalis, are maternal in genotype, but the important secretory and absorptive tissues of the placenta arise from the embryonic trophoblast and are of fetal genotype. Some known placental anomalies are genetic (Benirschke, 1965), and normal placental function is probably regulated in part by genotype. A. H. Schultz (1926) has shown that racial differences in face height, nose height, and nose breadth are detectable in Negro fetuses as early as the sixth month of gestation. If adaptations of Andean man—such as increased thoracic circumference and small size—are genetic, they might be found in the neonate (Tanner, 1960). A variety of mechanisms are thus available through which high altitude hypoxia could affect the fetus. These effects might be critical not only to the survival of the conceptus but also in terms of the total population increase and demographic stability of the high altitude population.

Observations in Animals and Man. During gestation the mother is supplying oxygen to the placenta and fetus as well as to her own tissues. The pregnant woman hyperventilates, and there is a decrease in the equilibrium level of carbon dioxide in the blood. The decrease of carbon dioxide is associated with a rise in oxygen pressure that facilitates oxygenation of the fetus (Hellegers, 1961). Increased heart and blood volume in the mother are further adaptations to the increased oxygen demands of pregnancy (Abramowicz and Kass, 1966).

The nonpregnant female withstands higher simulated altitudes than does the male. At all altitudes female rats have lower mortality rates than males, but this advantage disappears during pregnancy (Altland & Highman, 1962). Although altitude-induced erythrocytosis is approximately equal in human females and males (Berendsohn, 1951), there is evidence that altitude-induced cardiac hypertrophy is less pronounced in women (Northrup, 1960). C. W. Harris, J. L. Shields, and J. P. Hannon (1966) suggest that reduced menstrual flow in human females during the acute phase of altitude adaptation may conserve red blood cells; women express fewer complaints during this phase than do men, although erythropoietic and cardiovascular changes seem to show no significant sex differences during the first two weeks of altitude exposure. The altitude advantage in females may provide a reserve for the increased oxygen demands of pregnancy.

Maternal hyperventilation in pregnancy is reflected in the fetus. Throughout gestation fetal carbon dioxide levels are proportional to the low levels found in the pregnant mother. During birth the fetus experiences severe hypoxia accompanied by an increase in the level of circulating carbonic acid, but the neonate then corrects carbon dioxide level to the low value normal before birth. If hyperventilation of the pregnant mother is increased by exposure to hypoxia, the neonate will adjust his carbon dioxide level accordingly and will display a marked postnatal hypocapnia. Experiments in sheep and observations on Andean man (Hellegers, 1961; Gomero Espiritu, 1965) indicate that altitude and pregnancy are additive stimuli to maternal heart enlargement as well as to maternal hypocapnia.

The experiment of Moore and Price (1948) has been cited as evidence against an altitude effect on fertility. They did, however, report increased neonatal mortality and decreased infant weights for rats born at the 14,400-foot station. They attributed this to increased maternal cannibalism and decreased lactation. Other studies indicate that hypoxia may have a more direct effect on the fetus and neonate. Weihe (1962) reported a fourfold increase in mortality during the first twenty-four hours after birth in rats born at 3,450 meters (11,300 feet). A. A. Krum (Chiodi, 1962) reported that only 31 percent of rats born at 12,300 feet reached the age of six months. Hugo Chiodi (1962), studying rats born at 3,990 meters (13,100 feet), reported 35 percent mortality during the first three days of life. The mortality effect increased with increasing altitude; the mortality for rats born at 4,700 meters (15,500 feet) of simulated altitude was 80.7 percent. In pressure chamber experiments, 50 percent of embryos were born dead to pregnant rats exposed seven hours daily to 21,000 to 22,000 feet of simulated altitude (Van Liere & Stickney, 1961). Duane Johnson and P. D. Roofe (1965), using 18,000 feet of simulated altitude, also observed 50 percent stillbirths, reduced litter size, and lower birth weight. Surviving newborns had significantly increased red blood cells, hemoglobin, and hematocrit.

D. H. Barron and his coworkers (1962) examined the off-spring of pregnant sheep kept at the Instituto de Biologia Andina at Morococha, Peru, at 14,000 feet of altitude. They found no difference in weight or crown-rump length of the newborns as compared with controls born at sea level. Analysis of oxygen affinities and oxygen saturation of maternal and fetal blood showed that the oxygen pressure gradient between maternal and fetal blood at this altitude was approximately half that in the controls. Despite this, oxygen tension in the umbilical cords of the high altitude fetuses was normal. Barron concluded that modifications of the "placental barrier"—increase in weight and amount of surface area available for diffusion and reduction of tissue resistance to oxygen diffusion—must account for maintenance of a normal internal environment for the fetus despite reduced oxygenation of the maternal blood. Twinning was not observed in high altitude sheep, however, which indicates that there may be limits to the fetal mass that the sheep placenta can accommodate under hypoxic conditions (Metcalfe, 1962). The group of investigators reported local impressions that the human placenta is also larger than normal in the Peruvian highlands (Villee, 1960).

Toshiro Tominaga and E. W. Page (1966) have studied human placentas perfused with blood at different levels of oxygenation. In organs perfused with 6 percent oxygen for twelve hours they found dilatation of the fetal blood vessels in the placenta and thinning of the cell layer separating those vessels from the maternal blood. These changes make sense according to the Fick equation, which describes the rate of oxygen diffusion across the placenta:

$$Q = K \frac{A \, (Pm - Pf)}{D};$$ where Q is the quantity of oxygen transferred each minute, K is the diffusion coefficient for oxygen across the placental barrier, A is the effective area for gas exchange, (Pm-Pf) is the oxygen pressure gradient between maternal and fetal blood, and D is the thickness of

the membrane separating the two blood systems. The human placenta is evidently capable, if hypoxia reduces the pressure gradient to a critical level, of maintaining a normal Q through adjustments at the tissue level that increase A and decrease D. This adaptive response of the "fetal lung" parallels changes seen in the adult lung functioning under hypoxia.

It is not known if the placenta responds to hypoxia in this way in vivo, or if this response would ultimately involve macroscopic changes in placental anatomy. W. Aherne and M. S. Dunnill (1966) have found that the functional capacity of the placenta is related to the amount of villous or capillary surface area available for diffusion. Villous surface area is highly correlated (r = .89) with placental weight. A measurable increase in placental weight might therefore be expected to accompany an increase in the diffusion capacity of the placenta.

More recent experiments indicate that increased diffusion of oxygen across the placenta is only one of a series of adaptive changes that allow pregnancy to proceed normally in hypoxic environments. By using indwelling catheters in the maternal and umbilical vessels of sheep, J. R. Cotter and collaborators (1967) and E. L. Makowski and collaborators (1968) have shown that oxygen tension in fetal blood does decrease when the mother is exposed to high altitude during late pregnancy. Contrary to earlier experiments on altitude-acclimatized sheep, they report that the oxygen pressure gradient across the placenta remains approximately the same throughout the process of acclimatization. In six pregnant ewes transported to an altitude of 14,260 feet in the last third of pregnancy, Makowski and his coworkers found an initial decrease in the oxygen content of both maternal and umbilical blood. As mother and fetus adapted, the oxygen content in the umbilical vein carrying oxygenated blood to the fetus rose and reached normal values in all animals after two weeks. The increased oxygen content was due both to increased oxygen capacity of the fetal blood and to increased oxygen pressure. However, the increase in oxygen pressure in the umbilical vein paralleled an increase in pressure in the uterine veins. This indicates that maternal adaptations—particularly increased uterine blood flow—rather than placental adaptations were responsible for the improved oxygenation of the fetus.

Discrepancies in the results of these experiments reflect technical difficulties in measuring fetal oxygen tensions, but it is important to remember that many kinds of adaptations may be taking place in a single pregnant animal. Before reaching the umbilical vein, oxygen travels from maternal trachea to lung alveoli, across a diffusion barrier and into maternal arterial blood, then into uterine sinusoids and the intervillous spaces, and finally across the placental diffusion barrier. Thus, maternal adaptations such as hyperventilation, decrease in alveolus-to-capillary diffusion gradient, increase in uterine blood flow, and decrease in the affinity of maternal hemoglobin for oxygen can increase oxygen supply to the fetus. The fetus, too, can adapt by increasing fetal blood flow (Assali, 1967), hemoglobin concentration, amount of capillary vascularization, tissue myoglobin, and capacity for anaerobic metabolism (Metcalfe, 1967). J. N. Barker (1957) has observed increased production of Hemoglobin F in fetal and neonatal rats, mice, rabbits, and puppies exposed to pressure chamber "altitude." Placental changes may occur in addition to these maternal and fetal adjustments, and the specific character of a response may depend on genetic traits of the organism, the rate and degree of its exposure to hypoxia, and other qualities of its environment.

In comparing results of animal experiments and extrapolating them to the human case, it is important to consider species differences in length of gestation, fetal oxygen capacity, and placentation. Although all fetal mammals studied show increased oxygen capacity during the latter stages of gestation, particularly through production of fetal hemo-globin, only in man does the oxygen capacity of the term fetus exceed that of the mother (Kaiser et al., 1958). This may be due in part to the long human gestation period, but it may also reflect a relatively inefficient placental reserve in man, which shifts the burden of hypoxia adaptation to the fetus. However, placental size is much less critical in man than in mice or rats. In man placental weight accounts for about 40 percent of the variation in birth weight ($r = .62$; $.62^2 = 40\%$); the placenta stops growing between the twenty-eighth and thirty-sixth weeks of gestation, and during this late phase of gestation its nutritional capacity may become limiting (Sinclair, 1948a). In sheep the placenta continues growing throughout gestation, and never becomes a limiting factor on birth weight (McKeown and Record, 1953b). There are several other species variations: the histological relationship between maternal and fetal tissues is different in each of these species (Wislocki, 1929; Dancis, 1959); mice are born at a relatively earlier stage of development than man, and man at an earlier stage than sheep; term litter weight in the mouse is about 30 percent of maternal weight, while in man the term fetus and placenta amount only to about 5 percent of maternal weight. On the basis of these differences the effect of hypoxia on the fetus would be expected to be most severe in mice, intermediate in man, and least severe in sheep.

In summary, available animal evidence indicates that high altitude hypoxia has a critical effect on gestation despite the wide variety of buffering mechanisms present in the maternal, placental, and fetal systems.

THE FETUS

Before considering in further detail the effects of hypoxia on the human fetus and neonate, it is necessary to examine the still little-understood variables that control fetal development in the normal human case. These variables illustrate the secondary mechanisms through which altitude hypoxia may affect the fetus, and they would have to be controlled in studies aiming at demonstration of a direct altitude effect on human birth.

Most studies of the normal fetus have been devoted to birth weight. This is often the only information recorded for human births and is often taken as the final measurable expression of the complex components of the intrauterine environment. There is also a clinical motivation for studying birth weight. Seventy-five percent of neonatal mortality in the United States occurs in infants of low birth weight (2,500 grams or less), and the cause of low birth weight is known in only about half of these cases (McKeown, 1960; Griswold, 1966; Schneider, 1968).

Maternal Influences on Birth Weight.   L. S. Penrose (1961) has assessed the determinants of human birth weight as follows: (1) intrauterine and fetal environment, 30 percent; (2) maternal genotype, 20 percent; (3) maternal environment, 18 percent; (4) fetal genotype, 16 percent; (5) parity, 7 percent; (6) maternal health and nutrition, 6 percent; (7) sex of fetus, 2 percent; and (8) maternal age, 1 percent.

Table 1 illustrates the genetic data that formed the basis of Penrose's analysis of these influences. E. B. Robson (1955), in a further study of 205 cousin pairs in England, found a correlation of 0.14 for birth weights of children of sisters, but only 0.02 for children of brothers and 0.01 for children of a brother-sister pair. The important genetic influence on birth weight acts through the mother, and additional, largely unknown maternal factors account for almost 50 percent of the variation in birth weight.

Studies correlating birth weight with maternal height tend to confirm a genetic influence that acts through the mother (Hewitt and Stewart, 1952; Cawley, 1954). Tallness is known to correlate positively with social class, but even within each

Table 1. *Correlations of birth weight in related Japanese children.*

Pairing	N pairs	Correlation	Average overlap of autosomal parental chromatin
Half-sibs, one mother	30	.581	.25
Half-sibs, one father	168	.102	.25
Unlike-sex (dizygotic) twins	40	.655	.50
Like-sex (82% monozygotic) twins	220	.557	.91
Sibs, adjoining birth order	365	.543	.50
Sibs, one birth intervening	652	.425	.50
Sibs, two births intervening	151	.363	.50
Random Sibs (F = .003)	365	.523	.50
Sibs, parents first cousins (F = .0625)	440	.481	.50

Source: Morton, 1955.

socioeconomic class, taller women have heavier babies (Baird, 1964). Height is significantly correlated with pelvic area (Thomson, Chun, and Baird, 1963). Experiments in horses suggest that the mother is able to adjust fetal growth so as to make vaginal delivery possible. Foals produced by artificial insemination of Shetland mares grew to equal size at birth regardless of the size of the sire (Hafez, 1963). J. B. Bresler (1962) has found an excess of stillbirths and caesarean sections among short women. Dugald Baird (1964) reported a similar excess of caesareans among short Aberdeen women and conjectured that this resulted from genetically "tall" mothers, phenotypically short because of environmental factors, who were unable to control growth of the fetus to match their phenotypic pelvic dimensions.

Margaret and Christopher Ounsted (1966) have used a

measure of fetal growth rate rather than the crude birth weight to examine maternal control of fetal size. They studied a group of infants who weighed more than two standard deviations less than the mean for their gestation time. Mothers of these "growth-retarded" infants did not differ significantly from controls in height, but they did differ significantly in birth weight. According to the Ounsteds, mothers whose growth was retarded in utero tended to retard the growth of their infants. Furthermore, mothers giving birth to growth-accelerated infants—infants with a birth weight two standard deviations or more above the mean for their gestation time—tended to have been large babies. Margaret Ounsted hypothesizes that these individuals did not experience maternal control of growth in utero and therefore do not curb the growth of their own infants. She conjectures that the control is exerted by a chemical substance produced in the uterus.

Increase in maternal heart volume during gestation has also been positively correlated with the infant's birth weight. However, results are conflicting, and the correlation may result from the concomitant effect of maternal weight on both heart size and fetal size. The correlation between maternal weight and birth weight will be discussed in a subsequent section; several studies (Love and Kinch, 1965; O'Sullivan et al., 1966) report that it is highly significant. Mark Abramowicz and E. H. K. Kass (1966) suggest that the primary correlation may be between fetal size and maternal plasma volume—which is in turn correlated with maternal weight and heart volume. If maternal blood volume is low, the fetal supply may reach a critical level during periods of stress when maternal blood flow requirements are also high.

Maternal smoking during pregnancy was recently recognized as being associated with decreased mean birth weight. Nicotine has a vasoconstrictor effect, and smoking probably exerts its effect on the fetus by reducing uterine blood flow.

Recent studies by Joann Haberman at Temple University School of Medicine (personal communication) show that placental temperature decreases by one and one-half degrees after the pregnant mother smokes a cigarette. This decline in temperature as measured by thermography reflects decreased placental blood flow. Brian MacMahon and his coworkers (1966) compared 5,921 women who were nonsmokers with 6,180 women who had smoked during pregnancy. They found an overall reduction of birth weight in the smokers of 8 ounces (225 grams); mean birth weight decreased with increasing levels of maternal smoking.

The effect of cigarette smoking is quite large compared to other known factors. Males weigh about 120 grams more than females at birth; American Negroes weigh about 150 grams less at birth than American whites (United States, 1966); firstborns weigh about 150 grams less than later borns; and children born to staff patients weigh about 75 grams less than those born to private patients (Hendricks, 1964).

Lower birth weights in lower socioeconomic groups may be due to differences in maternal nutrition, which will be discussed in detail in a later section. Racial differences in birth weight probably involve both genotypic differences and differences in components of the intrauterine environment, but little comparative work has been done in this area (WHO, 1961; Abramowicz and Kass, 1966).

Racial Variations in Birth Weight.   Two general trends that have been used to explain racial variation in birth weight are illustrated in the studies summarized in Table 2: (1) birth weight tends to be low in races characterized by small adult size, and (2) birth weight tends to decrease within a given race from northern temperate to warmer southern zones.

The racial differences probably involve other genetic factors in addition to maternal size. A. M. Thomson and co-

Table 2. Mean birth weights by country.

Country	Source	N	Birth weight mean (grams) male/female[a]
India			
Madras	Theobald, 1965	29,775	2,800
Calcutta	Jayant, 1964		
Upper class		3,822	2,980/2,890
Lower class		2,279	2,590/2,500
Japan			
Hiroshima-Nagasaki	Schork, 1964	2,831	3,091
Equatorial Africa	Vincent & Ghesquiere, 1962		
Pygmies		31	2,607
Bantu		46	2,925
France	Ely, 1962		
Gypsies		44	2,837
French		100	3,326
England	McKeown, 1951		
Birmingham		11,152	3,400
Italy	Fraccaro, 1956	2,935	3,239/3,113

[a] Mean birth weight presented separately by sex if so calculated in source.

workers (1963) found frequency of low birth weight—the percentage of infants weighing 2,500 grams or less—no greater in Hong Kong than in Aberdeen (7.4 percent in both cities), despite the smaller size and presumably less adequate nutrition of the Hong Kong mothers. The flattening of the pelvic brim that Thomson reports in short Caucasian women does not accompany the short stature characteristic of Mongoloids. Thus, according to Thomson, short

Mongoloid women are able to deliver infants of high birth weight and do not need to curb intrauterine growth.

The low percentage of low birth weight among American Indians supports the existence of a relative reproductive advantage in Mongoloid women. The pattern of neonatal mortality may also be different for Mongoloids. Neonatal mortality for Japanese and Chinese in California is lower than that for whites (Rosa and Resnick, 1965), and neonatal mortality risk does not increase with maternal age in Japanese women as it does in Caucasians (Taff and Wilbar, 1953).

In contrast, individuals of Indian origin seem to produce small babies in Europe, Singapore, South Africa, and Rhodesia as well as in India (Tables 2 and 3). This disadvantage with respect to Mongoloids cannot be explained by differences in maternal size.

Africans also have relatively low birth weights. Custom and habitat undoubtedly influence these differences. The Masai, for instance, enforce a ritual fast on the pregnant mother during the last weeks of gestation (Roberts and Tanner, 1963). Malarial infection of the placenta may reduce birth weight by as much as 300 grams (Morley and Knox, 1960; Jelliffe, 1966), which may account for some of the low birth weight reported in the Mediterranean region as well as for some of the African differences. Maternal resistance to malaria may break down during pregnancy, and the infection can lead to reduced caloric intake and premature onset of labor (Thompson and Baird, 1967). Reduced mean birth weight has also been reported for women with the sickle-cell gene (Anderson et al., 1960). If this association is confirmed, it may explain the persistence of low mean birth weight in American Negroes.

Other Negro-white differences have been reported. Negroes reportedly have a low frequency of spontaneous abortions (Roberts and Tanner, 1963) and a high frequency of plural births—5.3 percent among the Yoruba in Nigeria (Morley and Knox, 1960), as compared to 2.6 percent for United States nonwhites and 2.0 percent for United States whites (United States, 1965; my calculations). Negro neonates are relatively more advanced than newborn white infants in terms of bone development and other indices of maturity (Schultz,

Table 3. Mean birth weights and frequencies of low and high birth weights by country and by racial and socioeconomic subgroups.

Country	Source	N	Birth weight mean (grams) male/female[a]	% less than 2,500 grams	% 4,000 grams or more
United States					
Whites	United States,	717,133	3,330	7.0	9.6
Nonwhites	1965	120,653	3,280	9.7	11.1
Whites	Meredith,	121,801	3,350	7.0	—
Negroes	1952	39,656	3,230	11.2	—
American Indians	Rosa & Resnick, 1965	—	—	7.8	9.3
Hawaii	Bennett & Louis, 1959				
Caucasian		7,055	3,364/3,246	6.2	7.3
Japanese		9,511	3,220/3,149	6.6	3.4
Chinese		1,760	3,238/3,147	6.4	3.3
Filipino		3,337	3,117/3,044	11.6	2.2
Hawaiian		297	3,272/3,200	9.4	7.4
Puerto Rican		685	3,239/3,122	10.2	3.7
Korean		436	3,276/3,175	5.3	4.3
England	McKeown, 1951	22,454	3,400	5.6[b]	9.1
Korea	Kang, 1962	1,489	3,658/3,606	9.5	7.0
Singapore Chinese	Millis, 1952[c]				
Famine[d]		4,571	3,080/2,980	8.5	0.6
Lower class		8,964	3,100/2,960	5.3	0.7
Upper class		298	3,160	13.7	1.3

Table 3. (*Continued*)

Country	Source	N	Birth weight mean (grams) male/ female[a]	% less than 2,500 grams	% 4,000 grams or more
Indian					
Famine		635	2,850/2,760	24.0	0.3
Lower class		875	2,960/2,900	14.7	0.3
Upper class		138	3,120	18.7	1.5
South Africa	Salber & Bradshaw, 1951				
European		1,757	3,410	4.2	8.0
Mixed		931	3,120	9.6	3.32
Bantu		7,611	3,090	11.5	1.86
Indian		1,738	2,950	18.3	1.6
Southern Rhodesia	Leitch, 1961				
European		736	3,320/3,240	6.7	4.2
Mixed		71	3,310/3,200	4.3	5.7
Indian		262	2,780/2,690	28.2	0.3
Nigeria	Morley & Knox, 1960				
Yoruba		2,973	2,820	19.7	0.3
Israel	Bromberg, et al. 1951				
Ashkenazi		4,179	3,210	4.6	4.0
Sephardic		1,303	3,180	5.3	3.8
Oriental		3,117	3,132	5.5	2.7

[a] Mean birth weight presented separately by sex if so calculated in reference.
[b] Excluded births under 28 weeks gestation. Other frequencies reported from England were 13.0 (Theobald, 1965) and 7.3 (Thomson et al, 1963).
[c] Percentages calculated by me.
[d] Severe food shortage in 1947.

1926; Meredith, 1952). There is evidence that African-born twins are at less mortality risk than twins born to European mothers; correspondingly, the difference between twin birth weights in Ghana and Europe is much less than the difference between singleton birth weights in the two populations (Hollingsworth and Duncan, 1966). The high frequency of plural births might confer some selective advantage on a rapid rate of fetal growth, since the more rapidly-growing twin has a greater chance of surviving the stringent intra-uterine competition and early delivery that usually accompany multiple gestation (Harrison and Weiner, 1964). The decreased gestation time associated with malarial infection is probably an even greater selective pressure favoring rapid fetal growth rate. Stanley Garn, on the other hand (quoted by Hunt, 1966), explains the Negro-white difference in bone development at birth as an adaptation of whites to the deficient sunlight of cold climates and suggests that light, slow-developing bones may be a favorable adaptation where rickets is prevalent. The association of rapid fetal growth with an overall decrease in birth weight in Negroes is somewhat paradoxical. Males, who have more rapid growth rates in utero than females, also have higher birth weights (Penrose, 1961).

Two kinds of study support the theory that ethnic differences in birth weight are based on genetic racial distinctions in anatomy and physiology. Table 3 shows the persistence of the racial pattern in groups from the same stem who are living in different environments and the persistence of racial differences in different racial groups living in the same environment. Data are barely available as yet, and some of the reported results should be re-investigated, such as Yung Sun Kang's (1962) report of very high birth weight in Korea, and Jean Millis' (1952) finding of a higher frequency of low birth weight among the Singapore upper class than in lower class births.

Other studies have shown that the optimal birthweight—that is, the birth weight associated with minimum neonatal mortality—is lower in Africans, Indians, and southern Europeans than in northern European populations (Fraccaro,

1956; Jayant, 1964; Hollingsworth, 1965). Millis' study in Singapore indicates that there are racial differences in the resistance of birth weight to starvation stress. It is intriguing to speculate that racial differences may also affect fetal sensitivity to other forms of environmental stress.

Racial distribution may account for the latitudinal association with birth weight. Osmo Koskela (1965), however, attributes the birth weight distribution to some direct effect of climate that influences the frequency of large babies. He found that 17.1 percent of a series of 15,147 Finnish neonates weighed over 4,000 grams, the largest percentage reported for any group. According to Koskela, the frequency of large babies decreases as one approaches the equator. J. S. Weiner (1964) cites the geographic distribution of birth weight as a case of Allen's Rule—the association of linear body build with a hot climate and stocky build with a cold climate. This hypothesis has not been tested: are the "stocky" cold-climate neonates shorter in length? What about birth weights in racial groups—American Negroes, for instance—who inhabit a continuum of climatic environments? Jean Millis (1957) studied 60 male and 76 female Caucasian infants born in Singapore—a warm, moist climate, near the world's minimum in seasonal variation. Birth weights in this sample (3,430 grams for males and 3,340 grams for females) were not significantly lower than those reported for Caucasians in cooler climates. Millis' data indicate that the Allen's Rule effect, if it exists, must act on populations over time rather than on conditions of the individual pregnancy.

In contrast, observations of seasonal variation in birth weight tend to support Koskela's explanation of the geographic variation as a direct effect of climate. Studies by David Hewitt (1963) indicate that the fetus, at all stages of gestation, is at greater risk of being expelled from the uterus in the summer than in the winter. He has found that the rate of spontaneous abortion and the frequency of immature births are highest in the summer months. He has proposed several mechanisms that might explain this observation: mothers are worse-nourished in the summer months; relatively more upper-class women give birth in the winter than in the summer. A study by the United States Census Bureau also reports a lower frequency of low birth weight—infants weighing less than 2,500 grams at birth—and lower neonatal mortality in the winter months (January to March) than in the year as a whole (United States, 1965). However, the difference is small, amounting to less than a half-percent decrease in the frequency of low birth weight. Thus, although the direction of the seasonality effect on birth weight supports a direct effect of climate on birth weight, the small magnitude of this effect supports evidence from racial studies that genetic and other factors rather than climatic influences account for the major part of the geographic variation in birth weight.

In summary, recent epidemiologic studies of birth weight tend to support Penrose's early analysis of the contributory factors. The racial differences outlined above probably result, at least in part, from differences in maternal genotype. As predicted by Penrose, general aspects of maternal health and environment, such as climate and nutrition, exert relatively minor effects on birth weight as compared to factors such as smoking and malaria, which directly affect the uterus (Mac-Mahon, Alpert, and Salber, 1966; Morley and Knox, 1960). Even the effect of maternal genotype on birth weight has recently been reinterpreted as a local effect which results from uterine secretions and which may vary in magnitude with conditions of the individual pregnancy (Ounsted, 1966). The influence of parity on birth weight—also mentioned by Penrose—may also be viewed as the result of a differential efficiency of the intrauterine environment. Thomas McKeown and R. G. Record (1953b) have found higher mean placental weights in later born infants than in firstborns (645 grams vs. 615 grams). As noted above, placental weight is highly correlated with birth weight—$r = .62$ (Sinclair, 1948a). Further study of the relationship between fetal and placental weights may result in more complete understanding of the birth weight differences found in epidemiologic studies in terms of local differences in the intrauterine environment.

The Clinical View of Birth Weight. The clinical view of birth weight offers the most useful analysis of the physiological mechanisms that produce observed differences in birth weight. Pediatricians define any infant weighing less than 2,500 grams at birth as a low birth weight infant with high mortality risk (World Health, 1961). Three types of low birth weight infants are recognized: (1) immature infants born before term, (2) growth-retarded infants, and (3) small infants born at term with normal proportions (Dawkins, 1965; Battaglia and Lubchenco, 1967). According to various systems (Yerushalmy, 1967), small infants are classified as "growth-retarded" if birth weight is less than the tenth percentile for their gestational age, or as "small-for-dates" if weight is less than the third percentile, that is, below two standard deviations from the mean for their gestational age.

Many female infants and Negro infants are of low birth weight, but they exhibit no signs of immaturity and no increased mortality. Placental weight is decreased in proportion to birth weight, but the ratio between the two weights remains within normal limits (Sinclair, 1948b). There is some evidence that infants of mothers who have smoked during pregnancy also belong in this category (MacMahon et al., 1966; Ravenholt et al., 1966).

Gestational age is calculated from the beginning of the mother's last menstrual period; forty weeks is designated as normal. Even when the mother's recollection of menstrual history is accurate, there is a certain amount of error inherent in the system (Treloar et al., 1967). The interval from onset of menstruation to ovulation is highly variable, and even if only the postconception gestational interval is considered, postconception "menstruation" occurs in a small percentage of women, and an unnoticed abortion may occasionally be followed by a term pregnancy without an intervening menstrual flow.

In the absence of an accurate estimate of gestational age —the usual case—the immature infant can be identified by lack of the testicular and breast development that occur late in fetal life, by immature neurological reflexes (Babson and McKinnon, 1968), by persistence of the downy lanugo hair covering, and to some extent by short stature, other anthropometric measures, and radiographic analysis of bone maturity (Ellis, 1951; Dawkins, 1965; Usher, 1966). Placental growth slows in the third trimester of gestation, so that the immature placenta is nearer its final weight than is the immature infant. The placental ratio (placental weight/infant weight) in immature births is thus higher than normal (Sinclair, 1948b; Hosemann, 1949).

Among infants of known gestational age, about one-half of those with low birth weight are mature in terms of gestational time, and about half of immature infants have birth weights exceeding 2,500 grams (Usher, 1966). The growth-retarded or "small-for-dates" infant may have normal anthropometric measurements but be associated with a disproportionately small placenta (Gruenwald, 1963; Tremblay, 1965; Wigglesworth, 1967). The placentas of these infants may also have more infarcts—small areas of necrosis on the placental surface owing to obstruction of blood vessels (Warkany, Monroe, and Sutherland, 1961). B. J. Van den Berg and J. Yerushalmy (1966) divided 9,199 singleton white male liveborn infants of low birth weight into quartiles that separated infants with rapid growth (weight gain/week of gestation) from those with slow growth rates. The infants with shorter gestation times had higher mortality, especially from respiratory disease, than those of equal birth weight but longer gestation time. One year later, the slow growth rate infants weighed 1.5 pounds less (P = .01) than infants in the rapid-growing group, even though mean birth weights were equal in both groups. Familial tendencies in maternal regulation of fetal growth, vitamin A deficiency, and chromosomal aberrations of the fetus have been suggested as etiological agents in growth retardation (Warkany, Monroe, and Sutherland, 1961).

R. L. Naeye (1965b; 1966; 1967) found greatly reduced liver, spleen, thymus, and adrenal weights in some growth-retarded neonates. Brain, pancreas, lung, and kidney weights were reduced, but near normal. The pattern of weight loss parallels that seen in postnatally malnourished infants. Myocardial muscle fibers are thin in malnourished neonates and infants, who have a relatively high risk of sudden heart failure. Many of these infants are hypoglycemic, which may be related to reduced stores of liver glycogen and to inadequate gluconeogenesis owing to the disproportionate reduction in liver and adrenal tissue relative to glucose-consuming brain tissue and insulin-producing pancreas. This pattern of reduced organ weights has been designated "fetal malnutrition" (Wigglesworth, 1967). Cell number is normal in these infants, and the pattern of reduction in cell mass parallels that seen in postnatal malnutrition. This type of "small-for-dates" infant commonly has placental abnormalities and is the product of a toxemic or a prolonged pregnancy. Naeye has described a second group of "small-for-dates" infants in whom cell number is less than normal. All organ weights in these infants are reduced, and there is usually evidence of chromosomal damage or of viral infection early in pregnancy (Naeye, 1966).

Recent research in biochemistry and epidemiology has been directed toward early differentiation between immature and growth-retarded infants. Mothers of preterm infants tend in the United States to be poor, Negro, multiparous, and anemic, and to have a history of periodic bleeding during the pregnancy (North, 1967). Mothers of "malnourished" growth-retarded infants often have chronic circulatory disorders—heart disease, diabetes, hypertension. If maternal weight gain flattens out after thirty weeks of pregnancy or if maternal serum estriol ceases to rise after thirty-two weeks, there is a high probability that the product of the pregnancy will be severely growth-retarded (Walker, 1967). Estimation of gestational age of the fetus can be guided by knowledge of maternal levels of certain enzymes produced by the placenta (Ischaliotis and Lambrinopoulos, 1964; Levine et al., 1966), and also by measures of biochemical maturity of the fetus, such as fetal serum gamma-globulin (Hobbs and Davis, 1967).

The clinical view, like the evidence from genetic and epidemiologic studies, emphasizes the complexity of the variables affecting birth weight. These complexities must be considered in evaluating and testing reports of birth weight depression in high-altitude human populations. Such reports have little meaning unless accompanied by information about maternal factors, such as smoking or race, and by additional data, particularly placental weight, gestation time, and histological study of the fetus, which can identify the type of birth weight reduction taking place.

Effects of Hypoxia on Birth Weight. Statistical evidence indicates that in man, as well as in animals, birth weight is reduced and neonatal mortality increased at high altitudes. The human evidence will later be reviewed, but first it is important to determine the relevance of the animal evidence to the human case and to analyze the altitude effect in terms of possible mechanisms.

The birth weight effect could be produced through the effects of hypoxia on the mother, which might either decrease gestation time or decrease the mother's ability to nourish the fetus. Or, oxygen lack could act directly on the fetus, retarding its growth. In terms of the clinical definitions given here, the low birth weight infants born at high altitude could be (a) immature, (b) small but normal, or (c) pathologically growth-retarded. Study of anthropometry, placental morphology, and causes of neonatal mortality in high altitude infants is necessary to identify the most important contributor to the low mean birth weights found at high altitude.

Each type of birth weight depression is associated with increased neonatal mortality, but infant viability can also be affected directly by hypoxic stress either in utero or in the neonatal period. Hypoxic stress during gestation may also produce long-term effects, such as growth retardation or congenital defects, which affect the individual's viability in childhood or adult life.

No change in the length of gestation has yet been reported for animals at high altitude, but there is a theoretical link between episodes of anoxia and the onset of labor. Monthly constriction of the uterine blood vessels, causing hypoxia, continue during gestation (Sinclair, 1948a). This, it is thought, may act together with hormonal factors to expel the fetus during the last week of the ninth complete cycle after fertilization. Theoretically, under the additional hypoxic stress of high altitude, the critical level might be reached during an earlier cycle. However, there is little evidence to confirm this theory, and Penrose (1961), in a study of 1,433 sibling pairs, found a correlation of only 0.15 between gestation times in consecutive pregnancies in the same woman. This would indicate that the relation between gestation time and length of the menstrual cycle is slight.

Blood glucose is another maternal variable that might provide the pathway for the altitude effect on birth weight. J. B. O'Sullivan and his coworkers (1965) have suggested that maternal prepregnant weight, more than age, parity, or stature, is the significant variable determining infant birth weight. The correlation between birth weight and maternal prepregnant weight was 0.19 in a series of 5,883 births (P = .01). E. J. Love and R. A. H. Kinch (1965) found a similar correlation in a series of 2,076 births—r was 0.21 for males and 0.30 for females. O'Sullivan and his coworkers report that prepregnant weight is significantly correlated with maternal blood glucose, the principal nutritional source available to the developing fetus. The partial correlation, holding maternal weight constant, between maternal blood glucose and birth weight was significant only in "prediabetic" women, who were defined as women giving birth to infants weighing 9 lbs. or more, who were 20 percent in excess of their ideal weight, and who were in the upper 5 percent of the population's distribution of blood sugar readings (O'Sullivan et al., 1966). Extremely high birth weight is a traditional diagnostic indicator of maternal diabetes; the excess glucose available in maternal blood, as well as hormonal effects, may be important in producing the large infant (Driscoll, 1965; Gruenwald, 1966). O'Sullivan's group speculates that the heavy or overweight woman, like the diabetic, supplies excess glucose to the developing fetus.

Rolando Calderon and others (1966) have studied glucose levels in acclimatized women at an altitude of 14,900 feet in Peru. They report below-normal levels in nonpregnant high-altitude women, and a proportionately lesser decrease in blood glucose during pregnancy at high altitude. Fasting venous blood glucose (mg./100 ml.) was 85.9 for 19 nonpregnant Peruvian women at sea level; it was 71.7 for 13 nonpregnant women at 14,900 feet. Twenty-one women at sea level in the third trimester of pregnancy had a mean glucose reading of 69.3; whereas the mean for 12 pregnant women at high altitude was 64.3. Numbers were small, but the authors attributed significance to these differences. Low maternal blood glucose might put an upper limit on birth weight, and the extremely large infants associated with glucose surplus might not be observed at high altitudes. Animal experiments have shown that a decrease in calorie intake increases hypoxia tolerance by lowering oxygen consumption (Newsom and Kimeldorf, 1960). The low blood glucose in the human high-altitude population may reflect a similar decrease in calorie intake, or it may result from altered glucose metabolism produced by altitude-associated changes in total body fat, acid-base balance, or adrenal secretions.

The role of nutrition in determining birth weight is little understood even at sea level. The association between birth weight and socioeconomic class in the United States (Hendricks, 1964) and the secular rise in birth weight observed in Europe, Japan, and the United States during the last century (Bakwin, 1964) suggest its importance. However, under near-famine conditions in Holland during World War II mean birth weight dropped only about 200 grams. Several studies (Keys, 1950; Abramowicz, 1966) report that maternal protein intake rather than blood glucose is the limiting nutritional factor in birth weight. Studies of nutrition in high-altitude human populations will be discussed later, but the incomplete evidence available shows no significant deficiency in intake of calories, proteins, or trace substances at high altitudes in the United States or Peru (Lichty et al., 1957; Baker and Mazess, 1964).

Another possible mechanism would act through altitude-associated changes in maternal blood pressure and uterine blood flow. McLaren (1965), working with inbred mice, found lower birth weights in members of large litters and in fetuses implanted near the cervix. According to McLaren, these effects could only be explained in terms of the local uterine environment of each fetus. Her hemodynamic theory of fetal growth emphasizes that the quantity of nutrients reaching the fetus depends on the local flow rate and pressure of maternal blood as well as its composition; McLaren also stresses the influence of placental size, which is controlled in mice by maternal blood pressure.

It is difficult to apply McLaren's theory to the human case. In man, systemic maternal hypertension is associated with small, infarcted placentas and with reduced uterine blood flow. Hypertensive women thus have a larger percentage of small babies; however, the percentage of large babies (over 3,500 grams) is also increased in this group (Gruenwald, 1966). Few data exist on the effect on birth weight of blood pressure variations in the normal range. Abernathy et al. (1966), in univariate analysis of 10,000 North Carolina births, reported that increased systolic blood pressure was associated with increased birth weight ($F = 23.4$; $P = .01$). However, they did not analyze this finding in detail, and their study did not include data on the placenta.

Armitage and his coworkers (1967) found no correlation between prepregnancy blood pressure and placental weight in a series of 900 births. They did report a negative partial correlation significant at the 5 percent level between placental weight and maternal diastolic pressure at delivery, which may reflect a tendency toward thrombosis of the uterine veins, retroplacental hemorrhage, and placental infarction and necrosis in women with borderline pre-eclampsia (Fox, 1967). From the available evidence it is difficult to predict whether the reduced systolic pressure and reduced incidence of hypertensive disease found in high altitude natives (Hurtado, 1960, 1964; Sehgal et al., 1968) have any consistent effect on pregnancy or birth weight.

Evidence indicating that growth retardation in fetal mice and rats results from a direct effect of oxygen lack on the fetus has been reviewed previously. There is no direct evidence as yet that the human fetus reacts to hypoxia in this way (Naeye, 1965a). On the contrary, Naeye (1967) reports that the pathological signs of prepartum hypoxic stress are only occasionally associated with the fetal characteristics of

growth retardation. A neonate with hypoxia displays pete-
chial hemorrhages, high blood lactate, amniotic debris in the
lungs, and meconium staining on delivery but usually has
normal cytoplasmic mass. Growth in the environment-depen-
dent stages of late gestation (Gruenwald et al., 1967) seems
far more sensitive to deficiencies in specific nutrients supplied
by utero-placental blood flow than to oxygen lack.

Effects of Hypoxia on Mortality.   Whether caused by lack of
calories or oxygen or by any other mechanism, a decrease in
mean birth weight at high altitude would probably bring
about an increase in neonatal mortality. Infants of low birth
weight—less than 2,500 grams—have low blood sugar and
albumin and are susceptible to convulsions and hypothermia
(McKay, 1964). If the altitude effect on birth weight involved reduced gestation time, mortality would be affected
even more severely than in the growth retardation case. Immature infants are highly susceptible to fatal respiratory
ailments (North, 1966). However, the association between
reduced birth weight and increased mortality is not universal,
optimum birth weight being reduced in some racial groups
(Hollingsworth, 1965). This may be the case at high altitude.
    Severe hypoxia, however, seems able to affect fetal and
neonatal mortality in mice independently of its effect on
birth weight (Johnson and Roofe, 1965). At sea level
infants who have experienced hypoxia in utero are usually
born asphyxiated and cyanotic, with severe metabolic acidosis
and elevated blood hemoglobin (Wigglesworth, 1964;
Haworth et al., 1967). T. H. Ingalls (1952; 1957), has done
extensive experiments on malformations induced in mice
exposed during fetal life to severe hypoxia in the pressure
chamber. Ingalls found that the type of malformation induced depended on both the gestational age of the fetus
and the severity of oxygen deprivation. About 60 percent of
the fetuses born alive to mothers exposed for six hours to

25,000 feet of simulated altitude had some type of congenital malformation. At 30,000 feet, the percentage was 79 percent, and at 35,000 feet, 87 percent.

C. T. Grabowski (1964) has suggested that hypoxia produces congenital anomalies by inducing generalized edema in the embryo. A 15–25 percent increase in water content was found in all chick embryos exposed for six hours to an 8 percent oxygen atmosphere. However, only one-third of the embryos died, one-third were malformed, and the rest recovered without apparent effect. Grabowski suggested that the differential response depended on the amount of disruption—cell distention, nerve and circulatory blockage—in the edematous embryo. Similar mechanisms may account for the variety of responses seen in mammals.

It is interesting that cleft palate, a malformation frequently seen in mice exposed to hypoxia, is never found in unexposed mice and has not been induced by other agents, such as nutritional deficiencies. Cleft palate is reported to be unusually common in both the human populations of Tibet (Ingalls, 1952) and Peru (Pereda, personal communication).

Naeye (1965a), however, has found no histologic evidence of oxygen deprivation in human newborn and stillborn infants autopsied at 10,000 feet in Leadville, Colorado. Douglas Grahn and Jack Kratchman (1963) found no statistical evidence for increased incidence of congenital anomalies at these altitudes.

Evidence on fetal hypoxia in man comes from studies at sea level as well as at high altitude. The classic view has been that the fetus lives throughout gestation "like a mountaineer" in a hypoxic environment (Barron et al., 1962). The newborn human infant, like other newborn mammals, is highly resistant to hypoxia. Oxygen consumption per unit of body weight in the premature human infant averages one-fourth that of the adult. In the neonate born at term, it is one-half the adult value. The adult rate is not reached until about three months after the end of the normal gestation period (Kerpel-Fronius et al., 1961). This tolerance has been interpreted as an adaptation to the hypoxic stress of gestation. Alternatively, the "tolerance" of the neonate to hypoxia can be interpreted as the functional inefficiency of the neonate's immature regulatory systems to operate at adult levels (James and Burnard, 1961). Whatever the efficient cause of low fetal oxygen consumption, it apparently has survival value. It is probable that even in "normal" sea level pregnancies the fetus undergoes brief periods of hypoxia in utero (Nesbitt, 1966). Some degree of hypoxia is always experienced by the fetus during the birth process itself.

As might be expected from placental and fetal growth patterns, the oxygen supply of the fetus becomes more critical near the end of gestation. Oxygen-carrying capacity of fetal blood increases in late pregnancy, as does fetal uptake of iron; placental area and permeability are maximal by the seventh month (McLaurin and Cotter, 1967). Walker (1959) found lowered umbilical-cord oxygen tensions in infants delivered after the fortieth week of gestation. Low readings were also found among infants of mothers with previous histories of stillbirths, infants with cord entanglements, and infants of low birth weight with the "placental dysfunction syndrome." Severely growth-retarded infants with signs of hypoxia have significantly increased hematocrits. These findings indicate that reproductive potential in women is closely associated with ability to oxygenate the fetus (Theobald, 1965). The results also suggest that excessively long cords and lengthened gestation time may be especially harmful if associated with the additional hypoxic stress of high altitude. Some investigators report that severe anoxic episodes during gestation or birth lead to hyperactivity and irritability in the neonate (Montagu, 1962). This is only one of many lines of evidence indicating that hypoxic stress during fetal life may have persistent effects.

At high altitude the neonate makes the adjustment to extrauterine life in a hypoxic environment unbuffered by maternal adaptations. The newborn child adjusting to the high altitude environment is not only a "small man," with many of the problems of metabolism and thermoregulation associated with small size, but he is also a man with immature endocrine and enzyme systems, with distinctive body proportions, and with low metabolic reserves (Dawes, 1961). The critical phase for the neonate is the conversion from placental to pulmonary respiration. Reported high incidence of patent ductus arteriosus in Andean populations (Alzamora, 1952; Marticorena, 1959) indicates that this conversion is not always successful at the low oxygen pressures of very high altitudes. Examination of 3,500 schoolchildren in Cerro de Pasco at 4,330 meters (14,100 feet) revealed 0.77 percent incidence of patent ductus arteriosus. Incidence is 0.1 percent in United States children, 0.3 percent in Lima adults—many of whom were born at high altitudes—and 0.05 percent in Lima-born children (Hellriegel, 1963). This shunt between the pulmonary artery and the arch of the aorta allows blood pumped by the right ventricle of the heart to bypass the still nonfunctioning fetal lungs (Patten, 1953; Potter, 1961). The vessel is usually completely sealed by the sixth to eighth week of life. Persistence of the ductus increases the load on the right ventricle, which must pump against systemic arterial pressure instead of against the lower pulmonary arterial pressure.

Persistence of the ductus is probably related to the elevated pulmonary arterial pressure that develops shortly after birth when the newborn is exposed to low oxygen pressures (Arias-Stella and Castillo, 1966). Low oxygen has a vasoconstrictor effect on pulmonary arterioles and leads to hypertrophy of the muscular media of these vessels (Cruz-Jibaya et al., 1964; Castillo et al., 1967). United States investigators report that pulmonary hypertension is more commonly seen as a complication of congenital atrial septal defect at altitudes of 5,000 feet than at sea level (Khoury and Hawes, 1967).

Hypoxia has also been proposed as an etiologic factor in hyaline membrane disease, one of the major causes of neonatal mortality. Sellers and Spector (1964) suggest that fetal hypoxia during pregnancy and labor increases capillary permeability in the fetal lung so that fibrinogen, normally not present in the lung, can enter. The fibrinogen then forms a coating over lung alveoli blocking gas exchange. Autopsy studies of adults who died of pulmonary edema at high altitude reveal a thickened alveolar membrane with a fibrinous encrustation like that seen in hyaline membrane disease of the newborn (Arias-Stella and Krueger, 1963).

Further studies indicate that hypoxic stress also has relatively severe effects on the postneonatal infant. Bone marrow activity must increase within a few days after birth in the newborn infant exposed to hypoxia (Reynafarge, 1959). Naeye (1965a) reported extensive pathological changes in the pulmonary arteries of infants and children autopsied at 10,000 feet in Leadville, Colorado. Anatomic evidence indicated that pulmonary hypertension was more severe in children than in adults. Abnormalities of the renal glomeruli were also found in the high altitude children. Similar conditions are found in children with congenital heart malformations or sickle-cell anemia and in newborn twins suffering the transfusion syndrome—uncompensated loss of blood to the sibling twin through placental anastomoses (Benirschke, 1961). The effects of altitude hypoxia thus seem to parallel changes associated with pathologic forms of hypoxia.

A study at 4,800 meters (15,700 feet) in Peru reported that at this altitude the heartbeat in the neonate was slower than normally observed. However, after the immediate postpartum period, values for high altitude infants were equal to sea level averages until about the age of four, when the low pulse rate and low blood pressure characteristic of the native adult appeared (Macedo Dianderas, 1957). Age-specific mortality at high altitude has not yet been correlated with these age-specific physiological changes.

There is evidence that low birth weight alone, independent of further hypoxic stress, has persistent effects on the developing infant. Subsequent low IQ and growth retardation have been reported for infants with birth weights of less than 1,500 grams. Since the incidence of low birth weight—2,500 grams or less—is about twice as high in the lower as in the upper classes in the United States (Griswold, 1966), much of this evidence has been criticized on grounds that the results reflect socioeconomic differences rather than long-term effects of low birth weight (Abramowicz, 1966). However, the finding of a stepwise decrease of IQ in each lower birth weight class and the observation of a specific detrimental effect on perceptual-motor integration rather than on the verbal skills, which are more highly correlated with class, constitute good evidence that there is a real association between low weight at birth and some type of subsequent neurologic impairment. Twin studies also report a deficiency of motor integration in the twin who is smaller at birth than his identical sibling. The mechanism of association is still unclear. Low birth weight may predispose directly to low IQ; both may result from pathologies of pregnancy; low birth weight and low IQ may be genetically linked; or prolonged hospitalization of low birth weight infants may lead to low adult IQ. Recent longitudinal studies have also reported that persons of low birth weight were still shorter and lighter at age twenty than controls of normal birth weight (Harper and Wiener, 1965).

E. M. Widdowson and R. A. McCance (1960) have produced stunting in rats by limiting milk supply during the first days of life, a stage of development corresponding to the last weeks of gestation in the human fetus. Weight and height were permanently depressed in these animals, and dental development, opening of the eyes, and puberty occurred later than in controls. It is not clear whether these observations are relevant to growth retardation at high altitude or if they are at all comparable to the human case. Firstborn children, whose low mean birth weight has been attributed to inadequate intrauterine environment, normally show rapid postpartum growth and have caught up in weight and height to infants of multiparas by the sixth month (McKeown and Record, 1953b).

Stunting effects have also been produced in rats by exposure to hypoxia, but many investigators attribute this to hypoxia-induced impairment of lactation rather than to a direct action of hypoxia on the fetus. In experiments with goats maintained at different oxygen levels during different pregnancies, J. C. Stickney and others (1962a) confirmed Moore and Price's earlier observation (1948) that altitude stress reduced milk yield in some females. They have also postulated an erythropoietic factor in the milk of hypoxia-stressed females. Stickney's group (1962b) reports that newborn mice and goats at sea level, when nursed by mothers receiving daily simulated altitude stress (16,400-19,600 feet), developed marked erythrocytosis.

A. A. Krum (quoted by Timiras, 1962) found that rats lactating at 3,810 meters (12,300 feet) produced only one-third the normal volume of milk. Fat content of milk was increased; carbohydrate content decreased. Krum attributed the increased liver lipids that are found in high altitude neonates to a "starvation effect" caused by lactational failure.

Other workers have reported that the infant weight loss and liver changes persisted even when rats born at high altitude were given nutritional supplements (Chiodi, 1962), which suggests that the hypoxia of high altitude acts directly on neonatal growth. In a long-term experiment with rats born at 12,470 feet at the White Mountain Research Station,

P. S. Timiras (1962) found normal birth weights and lacta-tion but an irreversible weight deficit in members of the F2 generation starting at the fifth day after birth. Virtually all of the F2 rats showed a doubled heart weight, increased hemoglobin and hematocrit, decreased storage of liver gly-cogen, and increased storage of heart glycogen. All these changes reverted to control values when the F2 rats were brought to sea level. The weight decrease, however, persisted in rats born at high altitude and transferred to sea level at six months of age. The growth curve for the rats born at high altitude exactly paralleled the normal growth curve, but with lower weights at each age.

In rats, brain maturation, as measured by response to elec-tric shocks, is delayed at high altitude. Neurochemical studies indicate that synthesis of neurotransmitter substances, enzyme activation, membrane changes, and myelinization are also delayed (Timiras and Woolley, 1966).

In summary, animal experiments at high altitude and ob-servations of hypoxia in human neonates illustrate a variety of pathways through which hypoxic stress during gestation can affect birth weight, neonatal mortality, and possibly the growth pattern and viability of the maturing infant. Further study of age-specific mortality in high-altitude human popula-tions is needed, as well as longitudinal studies relating birth weight at high altitude to the infant's subsequent develop-ment. Such studies would contribute to the understanding of both long-term altitude acclimatization and the long-term ef-fects of prenatal influences.

Several conclusions relevant to design and interpretation of studies of human birth at high altitude can be drawn from the foregoing review. First, although results are conflicting as to the adverse effect of hypoxia on fertility, animal ex-periments are in almost unanimous agreement that hypoxia—whether encountered naturally at high altitudes or artificially in chambers—adversely affects the developing fetus. Hypoxia has been found to increase fetal and neonatal mortality and the frequency of congenital malformations, and in some species it depresses birth weight.

In animal experiments there is an increase in the number of affected individuals with increasing altitude and a regular distribution within each population ranging from highly susceptible to highly resistant individuals. Available evidence from studies of fetal hypoxia in sea level pregnancies suggests that the response of the human fetus to hypoxia is quite similar to the pattern observed in animals.

The mechanisms through which hypoxia affects the fetus are still unclear. Experimental evidence indicates that hypoxia can directly affect cell composition of the maternal blood stream, the placenta, and the fetus (Berendsohn and Muro, 1957; Tominaga and Page, 1966; Johnson and Roofe, 1965). Ideally, all three systems should be examined, and histologic differences, as well as differences in crude measurements such as birth and placental weight, should be analyzed.

Interindividual and intraindividual variations in altitude response and in control of fetal growth are extensive. The only truly satisfactory way to control the many contributory variables would be to compare the same mothers during pregnancies at different altitudes. Exposure time at altitude must also be carefully controlled in order to separate acute from chronic altitude responses.

The theoretical understanding of altitude responses and of the factors affecting fetal development is still incomplete. Is there a genetic basis for the altitude acclimatization of native human populations? How close are the oxygen requirements of the human fetus to the functional limitations of the placenta? What are the selective factors acting on birth weight? Is high incidence of low birth weight associated with a general decrease in reproductive potential? Future research on birth at high altitude may approach answers to these questions.

Chapter II   Previous Epidemiologic Studies

Studies of birth statistics in the United States and Peru report that mean birth weight decreases and that neonatal mortality increases with increasing altitude. However, other characteristics affecting birth weight and neonatal mortality in man also vary with altitude, such as race, socioeconomic status, and availability of medical facilities. Existing studies have used various methods of controlling these variables, and the weight of the evidence supports a direct altitude effect. Many questions remain unanswered, however: does altitude depress birth weight by retarding fetal growth or by inducing premature labor? Does birth weight, like other physiological responses to hypoxia, vary exponentially with increasing altitude? Are there racial or sex differences in tolerance of the fetus to high altitude? The evidence bearing on these points is reviewed in the following sections.

MOUNTAIN AREAS OF THE UNITED STATES

Intensive study by the United States Public Health Service of 837,736 births in early 1950 showed that the mountain states differed significantly from other areas of the country. Mountain states—Montana, Idaho, Wyoming, Colorado, New Mexico, Arizona, Utah, and Nevada—reported a lower mean birth weight, a higher frequency of low birth weight (less than 2,500 grams), and a higher neonatal mortality (Table 4).

Race and sex differences were also noted in the mountain

Table 4. *Birth weight and neonatal mortality in the Mountain States.*

Study	Source	N	Mean birth weight	% less than 2,500 gms.	% 4,000 gms. or more	Neonatal mortality[a]
United States births, 1950	United States, 1965	837,786	3,320	7.4	9.8	20
Mountain States Births, 1950		33,625	3,240	9.1	6.3	24
Denver, 1953 (5,280 feet)	Lichty et al, 1957	10,566	3,035	11.7	3.3	—
Lake County, Colorado, 1949-1951 (10,000-11,000 feet)	Hospital records	577	2,655	48.3	0.0	49

[a] Deaths under 28 days per 1,000 live births.

states. Birth weights of mountain-state whites showed a greater depression from the national average than did those for nonwhites, but nonwhites contributed most to the increased mortality seen in the mountain area. Whereas white newborns were 130-200 grams heavier than nonwhites in other parts of the United States, the white-nonwhite difference was only 50 grams in the mountain division. The sex ratio of normal and low birth weight infants in the mountain area did not differ from the national pattern, but there was a difference in the sex ratio for neonatal mortality of low birth weight infants: the proportion of male mortality to female mortality per 1,000 liveborn infants of 2,500 grams or less was 235/131 in the mountain states, as opposed to 214/139 in the United States as a whole. Male infants of low birth weight were thus at greater risk in the mountain area.

It is difficult to assess the degree of these differences that is due to the relatively high altitude of the mountain states. Altitude of hospitals within the area varies from near sea level to 11,000 feet, and less than one percent of births in the area occur at altitudes over 10,000 feet, the threshold for major physiological effects of altitude (Grahn and Kratchman, 1963).

The nonwhite population of these states contains a relatively higher proportion of non-Negroes, especially American Indians, than is found in other states. American Indians have higher birth weights than Negroes (Rosa and Resnick, 1965), which may contribute to the decreased white-nonwhite birth weight difference found in mountain states.

The general decrease in birth weight is more difficult to explain. In the United States, average birth weight is higher in rural than in urban areas, and higher in home than in hospital deliveries, so that the low population density of the area acts against the observed trend. However, the percentage of plural births for whites is higher in the mountain area than in any other geographical area (2.14 percent as compared to 1.94 percent for all United States whites; P = .01). This difference would act in the direction of the observed difference in birth weight. Nevertheless, even if all of the excess infants of plural birth were also of low birth weight, this would account for only about 0.2 percent of the excess low birth weight actually observed in the mountain states.

As for the multiple birth frequency itself, available information indicates that the high rate reported in the mountain states is a local phenomenon, probably unrelated to altitude. James Metcalfe (1962) reports that twinning is quite rare in high altitude sheep in the Andes. Data from Peru indicate that multiple birth frequency is also rather low in the human population. The frequency calculated from the Peruvian census of 1963 is 1.3 percent (2,197/175,140) (Oficina, 1966). The Peruvian national statistics are incomplete and more heavily weighted with sea level births than are those for the United States mountain states. However, this frequency agrees with the percentage of twin births (18/1,481 = 1.2 percent) found in a series of 1,481 pregnancies in Huancayo, Peru, at 3,271 meters of altitude (Duda Vegas, 1962). Racial differences may influence the observed frequencies (Hunt, 1966), but too little is known about the causes of multiple birth in the general case to draw conclusions about the available data from high altitudes.

Coincidence of high dizygotic twinning frequency and low mean singleton birth weight, similar to that described for the Rocky Mountain area, is found among the Yoruba of Nigeria and among the Colombo and Ilesha of Ceylon (Knox and Morley, 1960). Among the Yoruba seasonal variations in these two variables are inversely correlated, highest twinning frequencies occurring in months with lowest singleton birth weights. Twinning frequency in the Yoruba correlates positively with mean maximum daily temperature of the fifth month prior to delivery and with daily rainfall of the eleventh month prior to delivery. These phenomena may not be comparable on a functional level with the statistical situation seen in the Rocky Mountain states, but the data suggest that a study of twinning frequency in this area should include analysis of racial and seasonal influences.

In 1957 J. A. Lichty and his coworkers reported differences in birth weight in hospital populations at different altitudes in Colorado. Data from this study confirm the trend seen in the census data (Table 4). Although one-third of the high altitude mothers were Spanish Americans, the investigators reported no significant racial differences affecting birth weight in the study population. Because of the severe climate in Lake County, people who live there tend to have jobs there; the socioeconomic level is thus relatively high. No significant difference in diet was found by the investigators between mothers having low birth weight infants and those having infants of normal weight. Lower birth weights persisted even in a series of 111 strictly defined spontaneous singleton births.

One hundred and twenty Lake County mothers who had delivered children at or near sea level before moving to the 10,000-foot altitude were interviewed about birth weights: 293 previous infants born at a lower altitude had a mean birth weight of 3,130 grams, and 261 infants born in Lake County weighed 2,840 grams—a difference of 290 grams. This comparative data, together with the elimination of race, nutrition, and induction of labor as factors contributing to observed low birth weight, make a strong case for a direct altitude effect.

Crown-heel length, head length, and head width were reduced in the Lake County neonates proportionately to birth weight. Lichty's group concluded that the size reduction was due to hypoxia. However, oximeter readings on the arterial blood of 142 Lake County neonates showed no overall depression in oxygen saturation. Hematocrit levels of the infants tested were also within the normal range. However, there was wide variability in both these measurements, and the investigators concluded that the size of the high altitude sample may have been too small to reveal real differences.

Douglas Grahn and Jack Kratchman in 1963 published the most recent review of the effects of high altitude on birth weight in the United States. Using census data from 1952 to 1957, they found a direct correlation between percent of low birth weight infants and altitude (Table 5). Growth curves of fetuses delivered at different weeks of gestation in the high altitude states and in Illinois and Indiana showed that the altitude effect became important only in the last trimester of gestation. This timing parallels that seen in the intrauterine growth retardation caused by racial and pathologic factors (Gruenwald, 1965; 1967). The birth weight difference represented a shift of the entire curve to lower values, not merely an increase in the low weight classes resulting in a

Table 5. *Percentage of live births at 2,500 grams or less by altitude interval, 1952-1957, Mountain States, white population only. Utah not included.*

Alt. interval (feet)	Mean alt.	Atm. press (mm Hg)	No. live births	% 2,500 grams or less
0-500	263	753	35,166	6.57
501-1,000	633	743	7,147	6.66
1,001-1,500	1,118	729	73,318	6.17
1,501-2,000	1,786	713	13,809	7.97
2,001-2,500	2,286	699	56,570	7.78
2,501-3,000	2,864	684	12,207	7.14
3,001-3,500	3,256	674	50,933	8.24
3,501-4,000	3,756	662	60,226	8.46
4,001-4,500	4,287	649	63,160	8.67
4,501-5,000	4,824	636	100,420	9.47
5,001-5,500	5,237	627	133,617	10.37
5,501-6,000	5,661	617	28,011	9.80
6,001-6,500	6,149	605	53,899	10.74
6.501-7,000	6,767	591	26,619	11.54
7,001-7,500	7,213	582	10,712	11.17
7,501-8,000	7,721	570	9,427	13.04
8,001-9,000	8,519	553	2,474	12.93
9,001-10,000	9,568	532	887	16.57
10,001-11,000	10,410	513	1,697	23.70

Source: Grahn & Kratchman, 1963.

bimodal distribution of birth weights. The 190-gram difference between mean birth weights in Colorado and those in Illinois and Indiana was highly significant.

The census figures, the detailed study from Lake County, Colorado, and Grahn and Kratchman's statistical analysis provide complementary views of the effect of high altitude on human birth weight. Together, they constitute good evidence that this is a real effect, and not the result of sampling error.

THE ANDES

Existing data from Peru support the association, found in United States studies, between altitude and frequency of low birth weight and neonatal mortality. In addition, the South American studies indicate that placental weight and the ratio between placental and birth weight may be affected by high altitude.

Richard Mazess (1966) has analyzed mortality figures from the Peruvian census of 1958 and 1959. He found that neonatal mortality (deaths during the first twenty-eight days after birth per 1,000 live births) in highland departments was 50 or 60—about double that reported for lowland departments. Using average elevation of the departments, Mazes obtained a correlation of 0.70–0.73 between altitude and neonatal mortality. Analysis of control variables—total death rate, post-neonatal death rate, and number of unassisted births—showed that only the first two were significantly correlated with neonatal mortality. Holding total death rate and post-neonatal death rate constant, the partial correlations of altitude with neonatal death rate were still quite high— 0.67-0.69 and 0.59-0.53 respectively. Mazess conceded that uncontrolled differences in health conditions and population composition may account for some of the association, but the parallels with studies in the United States suggest that altitude hypoxia itself is an important factor.

Data on birth weight in the Peruvian highlands come principally from unpublished theses written by medical students at the University of San Marcos. These data are summarized in Table 6, together with figures from the present study. Table 7 illustrates the altitude effect in terms of mean birth weight. The number of observations is small, and in most cases because of differences in study populations and statistical methods, analysis of their significance is not meaningful. The direction of the effect, however, is clear. In Peru,

Table 6. Frequency of low and high birth weights at various altitudes in Peru.

Source	Location of sample[a]	Altitude	N	% less than 2,500 grams	grams or more % 4,000
Oficina, 1965	All reporting hospitals, Peru	Various[b]	77,227	4.5	12.4
Acosta Chavez, 1964[c]	Lima (Maternidad de Lima)	203 m. (665 ft.)	—	4.8-7.0	—
McClung, 1966	Lima-born mothers[d]		326	6.8	11.6
	Cuzco-born mothers[d]		190	2.6	9.5
	Study series		100	5.0	7.0
Noriega Pinillos, 1961	Toquepala	3,060 m. (10,037 ft.)	309	7.0	—
Duda Vegas, 1962	Huancayo	3,271 m. (10,700 ft.)	1,500	8.9	2.9
McClung, 1966	Cuzco Lower class[e]	3,416 m. (11,204 ft.)	470	7.9	0.2
	Upper class[e]		155	11.0	0.4
	Study series		100	9.0	1.0
Alzamora, 1958	La Oroya	3,880 m. (12,726 ft.)	160	17.5	—
Sanchez Kong, 1963	Cerro de Pasco	4,340 m.[f] (14,235 ft.)	100	26.0	0.0

[a] Except as noted, all data are from hospital populations uncontrolled for mother's race, age, economic status, length of residence, etc.

[b] Of 175,160 births reported in Peru in 1963, birth weight was not recorded in 97,933 cases. Recorded weights are probably skewed toward higher birth weights because premature infants who died shortly after birth are not often weighed. Figures are also weighted toward sea level values be-

Table 7. *Mean birth weights at various altitudes in Peru.*

Source	Location	Range[a]	N	Mean (grams)	S.D.
Vilchez, 1954	Lima (203 m.)	2,500 g.+	490	3,612[b]	425[b]
Jara Velarde, 1961	Lima	1,500 g.+	100	3,297	511
Cuellas Huapaya, 1962	Lima	1,500 g.+	100	3,540	550
McClung, 1966[c]	Lima	1,000 g.+	100	3,300	544
McClung[d]	Cuzco (3,416 m.)	2,500 g.+	571	3,213	380
McClung[d]	Cuzco	1,500 g.+	619	3,127	472
McClung[e]	Cuzco	700 g.+	100	3,074	514
Jara Velarde, 1961	La Oroya (3,880 m.)	1,500 g.+	186	3,039	420
Sanchez Kong, 1963	Cerro de Pasco (4,340 m.)	1,500 g.+	100	2,730[b]	350[b]
Macedo Dianderas, 1966	4,860 m.	—	10	2,720	337

[a] Note differences in range. Peruvian studies compute mean birth weight from a set lower limit, which for purposes of comparison is followed here.
[b] Calculated by me.
[c] From study series. Includes all live births: twins, caesareans, stillbirths. Lower limit is smallest live born delivered during the study. The difference between Lima and Cuzco birth weights is significant at the .01 level.
[d] Recalculated from data compiled by Acurio, 1965.

---

cause hospital births are more frequent and records are more complete at low altitudes. Of the 175,000 reported births, 40,000 took place in Lima.

[c] Citing four studies from birth certificates: Llerena, 1935-1944; Villacorta, 1946-1947; Carrillo Gil, 1953; and Lara Cubas, 1955.
[d] From birth certificates, 1965 births.
[e] From hospital records, 1965 births.
[f] Native mothers at this altitude throughout gestation.

as in the United States, birth weight decreases with increasing altitude.

However, the increase in low birth weight with high altitude does not seem as steep in Peru as found by Grahn and Kratchman (1963) in the United States (Tables 5 and 6). The reduction in mean birth weight is also more gradual in Peru; it does not reach the value reported for 10,000 feet in Colorado until about the 14,000-foot level in Peru. Available evidence indicates that mean birth weight is about 400 grams higher in Cuzco (11,024 feet) than in Lake County, Colorado (10,000–11,000 feet). Frequency of low birth weight in Cuzco is about 10 percent, less than half that reported at comparable altitudes in the United States. On the other hand, sea-level birth weights seem roughly equivalent in Peru and the United States (see Figures 1-4). Possible explanations for this difference will be discussed in the next section; two obvious possibilities are racial differences or a more complete altitude adaptation of the Peruvian population.

Although Table 6 indicates that frequency of low birth weight at 10,000-11,000 feet in Peru is much less than that reported for the same altitudes in the United States, the reduction in frequency of very high birth weights is equally drastic in both highland areas. This effective disappearance at high altitude of the percentage of newborns weighing 4,000 grams or more may be a more sensitive index of the direct effects of hypoxia on gestation than are increases in the percentage of low birth weight infants. Little as yet is known about the causes of very high birth weight. Maternal diabetes is a well-known factor (O'Sullivan et al., 1966). L. S. Penrose (1961) suggests a familial basis for birth weights of 8.5 lbs. (3,869 grams) and over; in one investigated family, for instance, the mother had given birth to seven children, all of whom weighed between 5,897 and 7,796 grams. The altitude association, however, indicates that environmental factors are either more important than the

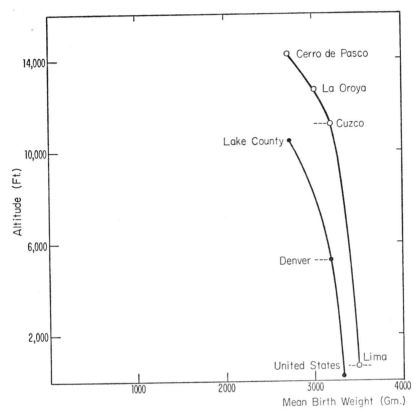

Fig. 1. Variation with altitude in mean birth weight in the United States and Peru.

genetic tendency for high birth weight or that they can modify this tendency.

One of the few published papers on birth weight at high altitude in Peru (Alzamora, 1958) reported an increase in placental weight as well as a decrease in birth weight, a high altitude difference that had not been mentioned in United States studies. Alzamora stated only that placental weights were "higher than normal" at the 3,880-meter altitude of La Oroya, but several student theses have presented quantitative

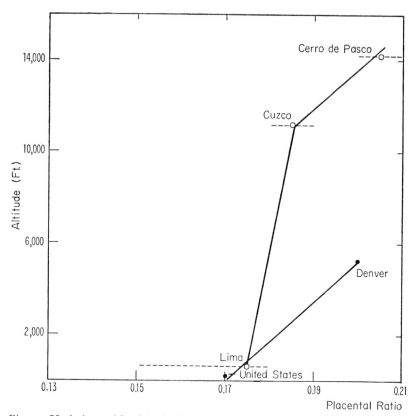

Fig. 2. Variation with altitude in ratio of mean total placental weight to mean birth weight in the United States and Peru.

data on this difference. Table 8 shows that the absolute placental weight reported by Sanchez Kong (1963) for his Cerro de Pasco series was no greater than that found in the sea level population in Lima. However, the weight of the placenta relative to the weight of the smaller high-altitude babies (placental weight/birth weight) is significantly greater at 4,340 meters than in Lima. Data from the present study, also included in Table 7 for comparison, confirm the findings of Sanchez Kong. Although there was no significant increase

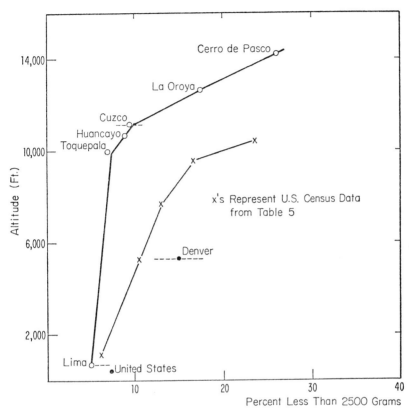

Fig. 3. Variation with altitude in percentage of neonates weighing less than 2,500 grams in the United States and Peru.

in placental weight at high altitude, there was a significant decrease in birth weight, and this is reflected in the significantly higher placental ratio at high altitude.

Placental ratio is the quotient of placental weight in grams divided by fetal birth weight in grams. The placental ratio is commonly used in South America and has been studied by several United States investigators. The textbook value for the ratio is 1/7 or .14 (Gruenwald and Minh, 1961). J. G. Sinclair (1948b), weighing the placenta without cord and mem-

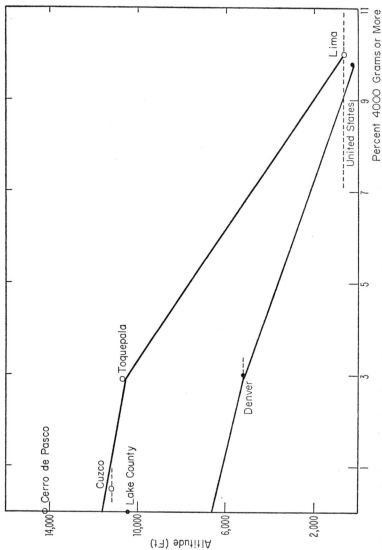

Fig. 4. Variation with altitude in the percentage of neonates weighing 4,000 grams or more in the United States and Peru.

Table 8. *Placental weight and placenta/birth weight ratio at various altitudes in Peru.*

Source	Location	Method	Placental weight			Placental ratio[a]	
			N	Mean (gm.)	S.D.	Mean	S.D.
Vilchez, 1954	Lima (203 m.)	+ cord + membranes	490	544[b]	83[b]	0.15[b]	.02[b]
Cuellas Huapaya, 1962	Lima	− cord + membranes	100	582	108	0.17	—[c]
McClung, 1966	Lima	+ cord + membranes	100	594	120	0.18	.03[d]
McClung, 1966	Lima	− cord − membranes	100	484	110	0.15	.03[e]
McClung, 1966	Cuzco (3,416 m.)	+ cord + membranes	100	596	100	0.20	.04[d]
McClung, 1966	Cuzco	− cord − membranes	100	503	92	0.17	.03[e]
Sanchez Kong, 1963	Cerro de Pasco (4,340 m.)	− cord + membranes	100	548	94	0.20	—[c]

[a] Placental ratio (placental weight/birth weight) was calculated for each case then averaged over the sample. See Table 6 for mean birth weights from these studies.

[b] Calculated by me.

[c] According to Sanchez Kong, the difference in coefficient is significant at .01; differences in placental weights are not significant; birth weight difference is significant (P < 0.01).

[d] Difference in ratio is significant at .01; differences in placental weights are not significant; birth weight difference is significant (P < 0.01).

[e] Difference in ratio is significant at .01; differences in placental weights are not significant; birth weight difference is significant (P < 0.01).

branes, obtained a value of .14 in a sample of 1,517 Texas births. Since placental weight is significantly correlated with birth weight ($r = .63$), a change in ratio does not automatically accompany either a change in birth weight or placental weight. In the United States, higher placental weights are found in later-borns than in firstborns and in whites than in Negroes (Hendricks, 1964; Toshio Fujikara, personal communication), but these increases are associated with increased birth weight and do not result in a change in the placental ratio. Sinclair (1948a) found high placental ratios among infants of low birth weight and suggested that these ratios might be a method of assessing "true immaturity" since the placenta reaches its final weight earlier in gestation than does the infant. According to Sinclair, neonates with placental ratios of less than .10 are at high mortality risk.

Placental pathologies illustrate that placental weight and area, and thereby placental ratio, can be altered independently of fetal weight. Increased placental weights are found in erythroblastosis fetalis and possibly in other conditions when the mother is immunized against a genetically dissimilar fetus (Kouvalainen and Osterlund, 1967). Heavy, edematous placentas are found in pregnancies complicated by hypervolemia or hypoproteinemia. Planimetric studies (Clavero-Nunez and Botella-Lluria, 1963) indicate that placental area per fetal weight is significantly increased in patients with uncompensated heart disease, but is normal in patients with compensated heart disease. Just as placental weight can vary independently of fetal weight, placental area may vary while placental weight remains constant or changes in the opposite direction; for example, although placental weight is increased in erythroblastosis fetalis, placental surface area actually remains less than normal. An effect of high altitude on placental ratio might therefore be the result of complex primary effects on fetal weight, placental area, and placental weight, and on the relationships among these variables.

In summary, available evidence from Peru thus confirms United States reports of a real effect of high altitude on the weight and viability of the newborn human infant. Peruvian data on the human placenta at high altitude provide a new line of inquiry, which may clarify the mechanisms through which altitude affects fetal development and birth weight.

BIRTH WEIGHT REDUCTION AT HIGH ALTITUDE IN THE UNITED STATES AND PERU

Epidemiologic studies of birth at high altitudes, like the animal studies, raise more questions than they answer. Reduction of birth weight is more marked in highland areas of the United States than in Peru; reduction in the percentage of very high birth weights seems to occur even at relatively low altitudes (6,000 feet), and the placental/birth-weight ratio is greater in high altitude populations. None of these observations has yet been adequately explained. The definitive test of the association between altitude and fetal development—controlled observation of the same women during pregnancies at different altitudes—has not yet been made. However, the similarity of findings on birth weight and neonatal mortality in the highlands of the United States and Peru indicates that despite confounding variables, the altitude association, together with the problems of interpretation that it presents, is real.

Differences in the severity of the altitude depression of birth weight in United States and Peruvian populations suggest that racial differences, the degree of maternal adaptation to altitude, or factors in the maternal environment may modify the effect of altitude on the fetus. Studies of Chinese and American Indian births (Millis, 1952; Thomson, Chun, and Baird, 1963; Rosa and Resnick, 1966) indicate that Mongoloids can maintain high birth weights even under adverse environmental conditions that depress birth weight in other races. There is evidence that perinatal deaths due to prematurity and to malformations of the fetal central nervous system are less common in Hong Kong than in England (Thompson and Baird, 1967). Hong Kong mothers also have a lower incidence of toxemia and eclampsia and have shorter labor. The Peruvian Quechua mother may thus have an inherent reproductive advantage over United States whites in addition to her possible specific adaptations resulting from more prolonged personal or racial exposure to high altitudes. No study has yet investigated the correlation between high altitude birth weight and the duration or efficiency of the mother's adaptation to high altitude. If the high altitude reduction of birth weight results from impairment of the mother's capacity to oxygenate the fetus, then a direct correlation would be expected between maternal circulatory adaptations to hypoxia and infant birth weight.

In addition to these differences in the Peruvian and United States populations, the Quechua woman in the Peruvian highlands is living in a much different environment from her counterpart at 10,000 feet in Colorado. Buildings are unheated in the Andean highlands, and women do most of the herding; they thus experience constant cold exposure as well as hypoxic stress (Baker, 1965). Low socioeconomic status is strongly associated with high rates of abortion and neonatal death in the United States (Hendricks, 1967), and it is difficult to see how these environmental differences would result in higher birth weights for the Andean women.

Furthermore, although preliminary studies (Lichty et al., 1957; Mazess and Baker, 1963) indicate that nutritional deficiency is not an important factor in either high altitude group, any nutritional differences that exist are probably in favor of higher birth weights for the Colorado women. A thorough nutritional study of natives at 4,000 meters in the southern Peruvian highlands (Mazess and Baker, 1964) showed that intake of calories, proteins, and trace substances was adequate by United States standards and higher than that reported at lower altitudes in Peru (Hueneman, 1954). Vitamin A was the only substance tested that was not present in sufficient recommended quantities in the highland diet. Vitamin A deficiency has been postulated as a cause of fetal growth retardation (Warkany et al., 1961), but because dietary intake of vitamin A is quite variable in Peru among villages and even among households, it is unlikely that this contributes to the overall difference in birth weight observed at high altitude. Since protein and caloric intake is more likely to be inadequate in the diet of semiacculturated city dwellers than of highland natives (ICNND, 1959), nutritional differences in Peru act to oppose the observed difference in birth weight.

Cigarette-smoking is the only major environmental factor that would lead to lower birth weights in the United States highland population than in Peru. No regular smoking was found among women in the Cuzco and Lima study samples. No evidence is available on the percentage of women smokers in mountain areas of the United States. However, in a 1964 study of 2,023 births in an urban county in the state of Washington, Ravenholt and his coworkers (1966) found that 68 percent (1,357) of the mothers were or had once been regular smokers. Children of nonsmoking mothers weighed 180 grams (0.4 lbs.) more at birth than did children of mothers in the highest smoking class (4,000 or more cigarettes smoked during pregnancy). However, sea-level mean birth weights are approximately the same in Peru and the United States, so that unless smoking increases with increasing altitude in the United States, or unless smoking intensifies the altitude effect, this environmental difference could not explain the observed United States difference in the slope of the plot of birth weight against altitude.

In evaluating environmental differences between the United States and Peru, it is significant that upper class mothers in Cuzco, whose environment most closely approximates that of the Colorado mothers, did not produce infants significantly different in birth weight from those of lower class mothers. Racial differences or differences in altitude adaptation probably account for most of the advantage in birth weight of the high altitude Peruvians.

Review of previous studies of high altitude birth points to a distinctive pattern underlying the reduction of mean birth weight with altitude. The decrease in the percentage of very high birth weights is sharper than the increase in the low birth weight class. The newborns are proportionately small (Lichty et al., 1957), and those weighing over 1,500 grams seldom require incubator care (Acosta Chavez, 1964). This pattern resembles the pattern seen in neonates whose growth has been impaired by inadequate intrauterine environment during the last trimester of gestation (Gruenwald, 1966).

Acosta Chavez (1964) has also reported an unusually high proportion of males among low birth weight infants born at 4,750 meters of altitude. Table 9 illustrates his findings as well as data from the present study. The proportion of males of low birth weight (males of low birth weight/total infants of low birth weight) in the United States is about 45 percent for the country as a whole and the same for the mountain states (United States, 1965; my calculations). The Peruvian data thus show a very low percentage of male low birth weight infants at sea level in addition to the high percentage at high altitude. Total sex ratio for all births did not differ significantly from 0.5 in any of the Peruvian samples. Although the high male ratio among low birth weight infants at high altitudes is statistically significant, the samples involved are small. Data collected in the present study came from hospital records and may merely reflect changes with altitude in the type of sampling bias. Perinatal mortality is generally higher for males than for females, and recording of birth weight may be significantly either less or more thorough for infants who die in the hospital.

Table 9. *Percentage of males among newborn children weighing*
less than 2,500 grams at various altitudes in Peru.

Source	Location	N	Male infants of low birth weight/all infants of low birth weight	% males
McClung, 1966[a]	Lima (203 m.)			
Lima-born mothers		326	8/22	36.4
Cuzco-born mothers		190	1/5	20.0[b]
Total		516	9/27	33.3[c]
McClung, 1966[a]	Cuzco (3,416 m.)			
Upper class		155	9/17	53.0
Lower class		470	29/37	78.0[b]
Acosta Chavez, 1964	Huaron (4,750 m.)	328	28/40	70.0[c]

[a] Data from hospital records.
[b] The difference between mothers giving birth in Cuzco and Cuzco-born mothers giving birth in Lima is significant ($P < 0.01$). Difference/standard error $= 58/19.1 = 3.0$.
[c] The difference between Lima and Huaron is significant ($0.05 > P > 0.01$). Difference/standard error $= 36.7/11.1 = 3.3$.

However, analysis of the data used in Table 9 in terms of overall sex difference in mean birth weight indicates that the overall male advantage in birth weight is also quite low among lower class Peruvians (Table 10). In the United States (1965), males weigh about 120 to 130 grams more than females; females are thus more likely to weigh less than the 2,500-gram limit of low birth weight.

This difference is said to account for the excess of females

Table 10. Sex differences in birth weight in Cuzco and Lima populations.

Location[a]	Population	N	Mean[b] (gm.)	S.D.	S.E.	Difference/ S.E. difference
Lima (203 m.)	Lima-born mothers					
	Females	148	3,257	312	25.6	
	Males	156	3,540	417	33.1	283/42[c]
Lima	Cuzco-born mothers					
	Females	86	3,499	330	35.7	
	Males	99	3,523	362	36.2	24/51
Cuzco (3,416 m.)	Upper class					
	Females	73	3,003	370	43.3	
	Males	65	3,388	445	55.5	385/71[c]
Cuzco	Lower class					
	Females	196	3,099	344	24.6	
	Males	237	3,174	370	24.0	75/34.4[d]

[a] Data compiled by me from hospital records for 1965.
[b] Includes only "normal" birth weights (2,500 gms. or more).
[c] Sex difference is significant at the .01 level.
[d] Sex difference is significant at the .05 level.

among low birth weight infants in this country. Table 10 shows that the male advantage in birth weight is reduced to less than 100 grams in the Cuzco population and also in the infants born at sea level to Cuzco-born mothers.

This overall decrease in male birth weight relative to female birth weight would be expected to reduce the normal excess of female infants of low birth weight; but the excess of males in the low birth weight group is still unusual. J. M. Tanner (1966) asserts that environmental stresses, such as malnutrition, depress male growth rate more than female growth. Altitude may act in the same way. The high mortality of low birth weight males in the mountain area of the United States (1965) may be a further indication of a sex difference in fetal sensitivity to high altitude. The whole area of sex difference in high altitude birth weight should be investigated in a large sample.

Related to the question of the mechanism of birth weight reduction at high altitude are the observations on placental weight in highland Peru. Fetal growth retardation at sea level is accompanied by a small, underweight placenta with increased infarcts and other pathologic traits (Tremblay et al., 1965; van den Berg and Yerushalmy, 1966). Placental weight is known to decrease with most types of decrease in birth weight (Aberle, 1930; Hosemann, 1949). Observation of decreased birth weight without decrease in placental weight at high altitude is intriguing.

Answers to these questions of the mechanism of high-altitude birth weight reduction could be approached by an epidemiologic study that considered variables in all three systems—maternal, fetal, and placental. Maternal smoking habits, race, parity, socioeconomic class, weight, height, and age have been correlated with birth weight (Abramowicz and Kass, 1966). There is much dispute about the relative strengths of these associations, but at least the first five can affect mean birth weight by 100 grams or more, and all should be controlled. Anthropometric measurements and other observations on the neonate can predict more accurately than birth weight the gestational age of the fetus (Usher, 1966) and could perhaps detect an overall reduction in gestation time or in fetal growth rate at high altitude. Although little is known as yet about the relationship of placental variables to other aspects of birth, Kurt Benirschke (1961) has prepared a standard protocol for placental examination, and data are now being compiled to determine normal limits of placental variation.

The definitive epidemiologic study of high altitude birth would also include a control sample, large numbers, and very high altitudes. The ideal comparison would be between the

Table 11. Birth weights of infants born to sea level natives (Lima) delivering in Lima, to mothers born at high altitude (Cuzco) delivering in Lima, and to Cuzco natives delivering in Cuzco.

Mother's residence[a]	Mother's birthplace	Female newborns					Male newborns				
		N	Mean[b]	S.D.	S.E.	Diff./ S.E. diff.	N	Mean[b]	S.D.	S.E.	Diff./ S.E. diff.
Lima (203 m.)	Lima	148	3,257	312	25.6		156	3,540	417	33.1	
	Cuzco	86	3,499	330	35.7	242/43[c]	99	3,523	362	36.2	17/50
Lima (203 m.)	Cuzco	86	3,499	330	35.7		99	3,523	362	36.2	
Cuzco (3,416 m.)	—[d]	196	3,099	344	24.6	400/43[c]	237	3,174	370	43.3	349/44[c]

[a] Data from hospital records, uncontrolled for race, duration of residence, etc. All women are "lower class" as defined by hospital status.

[b] Includes only "normal" birth weights (2,500 gms. or more).

[c] Difference is significant at .01. Note that this difference is in the opposite direction to the Lima-Cuzco difference because of place of residence. Cuzco women who have migrated to Lima actually give birth to larger daughters than do Lima-born women.

[d] Cuzco records did not specify mother's birthplace. However, of 60 lower class women in the study series giving birth in the Cuzco Hospital Regional, 18 (30%) were born in Cuzco and only 6 (10%) were born at altitudes lower than 2,000 m. (6,560 ft.).

same mothers delivering at different altitudes or, barring this, between groups of the same racial stock, one of which had migrated to a different altitude (Harrison, 1966). An N of over 1,000 would be necessary to confirm significant differences in sex ratio or neonatal mortality. Since other physiological effects of high altitude do not appear until the 10,000-foot level, this should be the minimum elevation of the "high-altitude" sample, and because acute altitude responses differ from those of acclimatized individuals, the high altitude population should be composed of natives. Such a study would be possible in Peru, where many highland natives have migrated to coastal cities.

Table 11 illustrates the possibilities of such a comparison. Analysis of the rough data obtainable from hospital records shows that infants born at sea level to Cuzco-born women have birth weights 300 to 400 grams higher than infants born in Cuzco. This fact, together with the other statistical evidence, strongly suggests a direct effect of the high altitude environment on fetal development.

Whatever its mechanism, the depressing effect of high altitude on birth weight seems at least as important as that reported for malaria (300 grams—Morley and Knox, 1960), cigarette-smoking during pregnancy (220 grams—MacMahon et al., 1966), or severe malnutrition (220 grams—Keys et al., 1950). Because of its association with increased neonatal mortality, further study of this type of birth weight depression has clinical importance, in addition to its importance for the understanding of physiological adaptations to high altitude.

Chapter III   Observations on Mothers, Placentas, and the Newborn in Two Peruvian Populations

Decreased birth weight at high altitude has been reported in several studies in the United States (Lichty et al., 1957; Grahn and Kratchman, 1963) and in Peru (Alzamora, 1958; Macedo, 1966). However, these studies have been criticized on grounds that observed differences resulted from variables other than high altitude—from racial or nutritional differences in high altitude populations or from differences in obstetrical practices or measuring techniques. Reports of specializations of the placenta at high altitude (Sanchez Kong, 1963) are similarly ambiguous because of differences in technique and lack of adequate controls. It is not yet clear whether low birth weight at high altitude results from shortened gestation period, fetal malnutrition, or a decrease in fetal growth rate, or whether the decrease in birth weight contributes to the high neonatal mortality, also reported at high altitude (Mazess, 1966).

The following study was designed to test these points in populations at different altitudes studied with the same methods. Maternal variables, placental dimensions, and infant anthropometry as well as birth weight were recorded for each birth. The aims were (1) to establish whether depression of birth weight is a direct effect of high altitude or an artifact of sampling error; (2) to assess, through anthropometric measurements, the maturity of newborn infants at high altitude; and (3) to determine which aspects of placental morphology are significantly different at high altitude. Because of the small numbers studied—100 births at each altitude—this is only a pilot investigation, identifying important variables that should be further tested in studies of larger samples.

STUDY POPULATIONS AND METHODS

Study populations were drawn from two Peruvian hospitals: the Hospital Regional in Cuzco at 3,416 meters (11,200 feet) and the Maternidad de Lima at 203 meters (665 feet) above sea level. The Hospital Regional is a modern hospital that was opened in 1965. There is one other hospital in Cuzco, the older La Lorena, which still has a larger patient turnover than the Regional. Patients say that they are not accustomed to the cleanliness and rigid scheduling in the newer hospital. The Maternidad de Lima is a much larger, older hospital with a daily birth rate of about 100, in contrast to the 3 births per day seen in the Cuzco hospital. There are several other maternity hospitals in Lima, and in both cities many women are delivered in their homes by friends or midwives. The general attitude toward medical care tends to be more sophisticated in the Peruvian national capital with its 1.5-million population than in geographically isolated Cuzco with its largely Quechua-speaking population of 60,000.

The base fee for childbirth is set by the government and is the same in Cuzco and Lima. A flat fee of 100 soles (about $5 in American currency) is charged regardless of the service required—caesarean, drugs, incubator care. This fee is low, even by Peruvian standards; $5 is about the weekly wage of a porter or agricultural laborer. The impression was that the Cuzco patients were relatively more prosperous than those in the Lima hospital. Cuzco mothers often said they had come to the hospital as a novelty "to see what it's like"; Lima mothers often said they came because they did not know or could not afford a midwife. Fewer than 10 percent of the lower class women in either sample had received any prenatal care. "Upper class" women included in the Cuzco sample paid a daily hospital rate of from $5 to $10 plus a private doctor's fee.

In both hospitals the study sample was unselected and included all live births within a defined time interval. In Cuzco, because of the limited number of births and time limitations, it was necessary to include upper class births, twins, immature infants, and caesarean sections in order to make up an adequate sample. A similar method was followed in Lima; all births occurring between 8 and 10 P.M. each evening were included in the sample up to an N of 100. For purposes of analysis, twins, immatures, and caesareans were removed from both groups, "upper class" births from the Cuzco sample, and Negroids and Asiatics (Peruvian Chinese) from the Lima sample.

Weights were taken at birth by myself or by trained hospital personnel. Measurements of infant lengths, circumferences, and skinfolds were taken within twelve hours of birth. Infants under incubator care were not measured. Total length and crown-rump length were taken with the infant extended on a measuring board. Head and chest circumferences and arm length were measured with a steel tape (Garn and Shamir, 1958). Skinfolds were taken with the Lange skinfold caliper at eight sites: throat on the midline beneath the chin; forearm, lateral to cubital fossa with elbow flexed 90 degrees; upper arm, midway from acromion to olecranon; chest 1, juxta nipple, with caliper in line with the anterior of the axilla; chest 2, on the midaxillary line at the level of the xiphoid process; back, immediately below the inferior angle of the scapula; waist, about 5 cm. lateral to the umbilicus; and calf, lateral to the popliteal fossa, thigh horizontal and leg vertical (Baker, Hunt, and Sen, 1958; Baker, 1959).

The placenta was examined within eight hours of birth; placentas were kept refrigerated in metal containers. According to Kurt Benirschke (1961; 1965), no significant change in placental weight or consistency should take place during this interval. The placental examination followed the protocol developed by Benirschke (1961) (see Appendix I).

Mothers were interviewed and measured on the first postpartum day, and early release plus lack of co-operation—particularly refusal to submit to the anthropometer or skinfold calipers—caused loss of some mothers from the sample. Standing height was measured with the anthropometer, weight in kilograms with balance scales, and eight skinfolds were taken by the method described above for the infant. Information on reproductive history was taken by the author in Spanish or Quechua; each child was named in order and carefully discussed, in addition to intervening abortions or stillbirths.

Each mother was rated by the author for race on a scale from 1 to 5, 1 being most Indian in appearance and 5 being most European. Ratings were given on the basis of skin color, facial features, amount of body hair, and texture and straightness of hair. Neither class 1 nor class 5 represents a "pure" type. There is a long history of racial mixing in Peru, and racial classification by Peruvians is more directly related to economic status and to life style than to biologic differences. In this study the women classified as mostly Indian (classes 1 and 2) were more fluent in Quechua, less fluent in Spanish, had received fewer years of schooling, and had been born at higher altitudes than those ranked as mostly European (classes 4 and 5). Stature correlated with racial classification at the .05 level, the more European women being taller.

Additional data on birth weight were obtained from hospital records of 1965 births. Cuzco pediatricians were interested in birth weight, and the hospital had kept complete records of infants born in 1965. In Lima, copies of the birth certificates of all 1965 births were available. Birth weight was often omitted on the birth certificate, and weights were probably not as accurate as those taken by trained Cuzco personnel. The mother's birthplace was recorded in Lima, but not on the Cuzco hospital records.

Table 12 shows the general pattern of differences in the

Table 12. Dimensions of the neonate and the placenta at high altitude (Cuzco) and at sea level (Lima).

	Cuzco		Lima	
Variable[a]	Mean	S.D.	Mean	S.D.
Birth weight (gm.)[b]	3,092.8	457.6	3,311.5	479.6
Infant length (cm.)[c,d]	49.6	1.6	48.9	1.8
Crown-rump length (cm.)[b,d]	32.1	1.4	33.2	1.4
Thoracic circumference (cm.)[c,d]	32.6	1.4	33.2	1.9
Arm length (cm.)[b,d]	19.5	1.0	20.2	1.0
Mean skinfold (8 sites; mm.)[c,d]	4.4	0.9	4.7	0.9
Placental weight/birth weight ratio[b,e]	.17	.03	.15	.03
Minimum placental diameter (cm.)[c]	16.2	1.7	15.7	1.7
Placental depth (cm.)[b]	2.2	0.4	2.5	0.5
Cord length (cm.)[b]	43.9	11.4	49.7	9.8
Number of placental infarcts per placenta[c]	0.9	1.2	0.4	0.8
Percentage of placentas in sample with one or more infarcts[b]	53%		31%	

[a] Corrected populations. "Normal" births to lower-class mestizo mothers. N = 73 in Cuzco, 88 in Lima.

[b] $P < .01$. Difference/standard error of difference = 2.5 or greater.

[c] $P < .05$. Difference/standard error of difference = 2 to 2.5.

[d] Lengths, circumferences, and skinfolds were taken on only 68 of the Cuzco infants and 85 of the Lima infants.

[e] The Benirshke placental weight, which is the weight of the body of the placenta alone, after cord and membrances have been cut, was used in calculating this ratio.

newborn infant and placenta at high altitude. At 11,000 feet of altitude the neonate was more than 200 grams lighter than the sea level infant. Although his head circumference and total length were not reduced (total length was in fact increased significantly—P = 5 percent—in Cuzco infants, trunk length, chest circumference, and arm length were slightly less than the mean values for sea level infants. Skinfolds were also slightly reduced at high altitude. The placenta, however, was not reduced in weight at high altitude, and this was reflected in a higher placental weight/birth weight ratio in the Cuzco population. The relative increase in placental weight at high altitude was apparently accompanied by an absolute increase in placental area. The maximum diameter in Cuzco was slightly but not significantly larger (18.6 cm. as opposed to 18.3 cm. in Lima), and the minimum diameter was significantly larger than the sea level mean. The placenta was also slightly flattened and more likely to be infarcted at high altitude, and the umbilical cord was relatively short.

BIRTH WEIGHT AS EVIDENCE FOR
DIRECT ALTITUDE EFFECT

The decrease in mean birth weight at the Cuzco altitude is highly significant statistically. The problem in previous studies has been to prove that the difference is attributable to altitude itself rather than to other factors only secondarily associated with altitude. Table 13 lists factors that have been associated with birth weight in previous studies.

In addition to being questioned about smoking, mothers in the sample were asked if they chewed coca leaves. The effect of cocaine on birth weight is not known, but since coca use is more common at high altitudes, it may have contributed to differences observed in previous Peruvian studies. However, none of the mothers in these two samples used coca, so this factor did not affect the observed birth weight difference in this study.

It is possible that two or more of the listed variables could

Table 13. *Comparability of the high altitude (Cuzco) and sea level (Lima) mothers in respect to factors other than altitude that may influence birth weight.*

Variable[a]	Cuzco Mean	Cuzco S.D.	Lima Mean	Lima S.D.
Maternal factors	N = 60		N = 83	
Smoking	0.0	0.0	0.0	0.0
Race[b,c]	1.9	1.0	2.5	0.9
Parity	3.3	2.6	3.7	3.0
Postpartum weight (kg.)	54.6	6.8	54.7	6.8
Stature (cm.)	148.7	4.9	147.1	4.6
Skinfolds[d]				
Triceps (mm.)[b]	16.9	4.3	13.5	3.8
Subscapular (mm.)	18.1	4.7	17.8	5.3
Mean (8 sites; mm.)	13.7	2.8	13.0	3.0
Age (yr.)	25.2	6.3	25.6	6.4
Percentage primiparas	20/60 = 33.3%		22/83 = 26.5%	
Sex of infant	N = 73		N = 88	
Percentage males	38/73 = 52%		51/88 = 58%	

[a] Corrected samples. "Normal" births to lower-class mestizo mothers.

[b] $P < .01$. Other variables are not significantly different.

[c] See text for definition of racial categories. Category 1 is more Indian, less Spanish phenotypically than category 2. Although statistically significant, this difference may have little biological significance.

[d] Maternal skinfolds have not been directly correlated with infant birth weights. However, they are an index of maternal nutrition, which influences birth weight (Keys et al., 1950).

have combined to produce the observed difference. However, race and triceps skinfold are the only maternal factors listed that differed significantly between the populations. The difference in triceps skinfold is in the direction of higher values in Cuzco, precisely the opposite of what would be expected if the Cuzco mothers were worse-nourished.

"Racial" difference is difficult to assess. Mestizos of Classes 2 and 3 differ little in appearance. Further, Table 11 shows that Cuzco-born women in Lima gave birth to infants that were no lighter in weight than infants of the probably more European Lima-born mothers, but which were significantly heavier than babies born in Cuzco. This is good evidence that the altitude-associated difference in racial composition did not contribute significantly to the observed altitude difference in birth weight. The observation that in Cuzco birth weight was also depressed among the more European upper class infants (Table 10) is further evidence for a direct altitude effect. Of course, the only really satisfactory control of the genetic factors affecting birth weight would be comparison of consecutive gestations in the same mother at different altitudes. Lichty and his coworkers (1957) have made such a study among Colorado women and report that a 300-gram difference between high altitude (10,000 feet) and sea-level birth weights persisted in the genetically controlled sample.

More effective altitude adaptation of the mother is one possible explanation for the lesser depression of birth weight in this Peruvian sample than was found at similar altitudes in Colorado (Grahn and Kratchman, 1963). Only 6 (10 percent) of the mothers in the Cuzco sample had been born at altitudes of less than 2,000 meters (6,400 feet). Only three had come to Cuzco from sea level altitudes during the pregnancy; they gave birth to infants weighing 2,310, 2,650, and 2,840 grams. This very small sample gives some support to the hypothesis that birth weight depression is less severe in the better-adapted mothers.

Table 13 shows that the Lima group contained a slightly higher percentage of males and later-born infants than did the Cuzco sample. Although neither difference was significant, both differences are in the direction of higher birth weights for the Lima sample (Tables 14 and 15). In order to test the effect of these differences on the observed difference in birth weight, expected mean birth weights were calculated for a hypothetical Cuzco population containing 58 percent

Table 14. Mean birth and placental weights by sex of infant and mother's parity, among lower class Negroes and whites in the United States.

Sample	Birth weight (gm.)		Placental weight (gm.)[a]	
	Firstborn	Later born	Firstborn	Later born
Negroes				
Males	N = 382	N = 1402		
	2,905	3,158	542	581
Females	N = 392	N = 1327		
	2,854	3,045	541	577
Whites				
Males	N = 42	N = 141		
	3,212	3,309	577	599
Females	N = 37	N = 137		
	3,042	3,248	572	599

Source: Hendricks, 1964.
[a] Total placental weight, including cord and membranes.

rather than 52 percent males and for a Cuzco population containing 27 percent rather than 33 percent firstborns. It was found that the slight excess of females in Cuzco depressed mean birth weight by only 5 grams (expected = 3,096.7; actual = 3,092.8), and the slight excess of firstborns affected the means by less than 15 grams (expected = 3,104.7; actual = 3,092.8). An increase of even 20 grams in the Cuzco mean birth weight would not have affected the significance of the difference between the Cuzco and Lima means. The actual difference was 219 grams, with a standard error of 77. A 190-gram difference in birth weight would still be significant at the .01 level, and even a 150-gram difference would be significant at .05. The fact that significant differences in birth weights were also found in the larger samples taken from hospital records (Table 11) is further evidence that the

Table 15. Birth weight, placental weight, and the coefficient of correlation between them by sex of infant and mother's parity, among lower class mestizos in Lima and Cuzco.

	Cuzco			Lima		
Sample[a]	Birth weight (gm.)	Placental weight (gm.)[b]	r[c]	Birth weight (gm.)	Placental weight (gm.)	r[c]
Males[2]	N = 38			N = 51		
Mean	3,130	606	.58	3,290	584	.61
S.D.	458	95		477	102	
Females	N = 35			N = 37		
Mean	3,053	601	.66	3,342	604	.60
S.D.	425	98		488	136	
Firstborns	N = 20			N = 22		
Mean	2,897	580	.78	3,207	578	.45
S.D.	444	92		398	101	
Later borns	N = 40			N = 61		
Mean	3,206.6	609	.51	3,348	599	.64
S.D.	371	101		516	125	

[a] This table is not strictly comparable to Table 14. Because of the small numbers (the male-firstborn category in Cuzco, for instance, would have contained only ten individuals), breakdowns have been made separately by sex of infant and by mother's parity.

[b] Total placental weight, including cord and membranes. This weight is about 100 grams more than the Benirschke-method placental weight used to calculate the placental ratio in Table 12.

[c] $P < .01$. Because of the small N's, significance tests on the means are not presented.

difference found in the study populations was not produced by sampling error.

Tables 14 and 15 illustrate some intriguing characteristics of the high altitude sample that should be further investigated in larger populations. The high percentage of males among infants of low birth weight at high altitude and the apparently reduced male advantage in birth weight in Mestizo populations have been illustrated in Tables 9 and 10 for larger Peruvian samples. In the small study sample Cuzco males outweighed the females by less than 100 grams, and the Lima females were actually heavier than males.

In Cuzco mean weight for firstborns was 310 grams less than the mean for later born children; this compares with a 150-gram difference between first- and later-borns in Lima, and to differences of 100-200 grams reported among American whites. Clearly the numbers are too small to demonstrate real differences among these populations. However, the high correlation between birth weight and placental weight in the Cuzco firstborns is a further indication that altitude effects may be more critical for these than for later-born children.

Table 14 and 15 also illustrate the unique relationship between birth and placental weight in the Cuzco population. Birth and placental weights are roughly equal in Lima Mestizos and United States whites. Mean birth weight in both Cuzco Mestizos and United States Negroes is diminished by about 200 grams, but whereas Negro placental weights are proportionately diminished, placental weights in Cuzco remain unchanged from sea level values.

Birth weight was positively correlated at both altitudes with placental weight and with infant dimensions (Table 16). Of the measured maternal dimensions, only the mother's weight correlated significantly with birth weight. Birth weight was negatively correlated with the placental ratio; that is, the smaller infants tended to have more placental weight per unit body weight. Sinclair (1948b) attributes this to the relatively early maturation of the placenta as compared to the fetus and suggests that a high placental ratio is an indicator of relative immaturity of the infant. P. Armitage and his co-workers (1967) report that placental weight is negatively correlated with length of gestation (-0.612) but positively correlated with infant weight (0.122); the negative correlation found in my study between birth weight and placental ratio is another expression of these relationships.

Table 16. Variables correlating significantly with birth weight in the Cuzco and Lima samples.

Variable	Cuzco sample		Lima sample	
	N	r[a]	N	r[a]
Mother's postpartum weight	56	.35	88	.27[b,c]
Placental ratio[d]				
(placental weight/birth weight)	73	—.41	88	—.14[e]
Placental weight[d]	73	.58	88	.59
Maximum diameter[f]	73	.44	88	.43
Minimum diameter[f]	73	.24	88	.48
Maximum depth[f]	73	.07[e]	88	.22
Infant length[g]	68	.74	85	.71
Crown-rump length	68	.75	85	.68
Head circumference	68	.62	85	.72
Thoracic circumference	68	.83	85	.84
Arm length	68	.37	85	.55
Skinfolds				
Triceps	68	.41	85	.45
Subscapular	68	.42	85	.58
Mean (8 sites)	68	.50	85	.66

[a] $P < .01$ (except as noted).
[b] The only maternal variable that correlated significantly with birth weight.
[c] $P < .05$.
[d] Taken by the Benirschke method, with cord and membranes cut.
[e] P not significant.
[f] Holding placental weight constant, the partial correlation of each of these variables with birth weight was not significant.
[g] All infant measurements were highly intercorrelated; only the general relation of infant dimensions to birth weight is treated here.

DIMENSIONS AND MATURITY OF NEONATE

What causes the reduced mean birth weight observed at high altitude? Increased incidence of premature labor, such as is found in malarial regions? Increased incidence of fetal malnutrition, such as occurs in the placental dysfunction syndrome? Decreased fetal growth rate, such as that found in female relative to male infants? Several possible explanations can be eliminated by analysis of the data collected in this study, but no single unambiguous answer emerges.

No bimodality was detected in any measured variable of the high altitude neonate. For example, the increased percentage of low birth weight infants at high altitude was not an independent phenomenon but was accompanied by disappearance of the very high birth weights no longer within the high altitude range (Grahn and Kratchman, 1963). The altitude effect must therefore act on the population as a whole and not on any specific subgroup. The birth weight depression might reflect an overall decrease in mean gestation time or in maternal nutritional or oxygenation capacity, but it could not be produced by, for example, an increase in the percentage of women with severe malnutrition or with pathologic conditions leading to early onset of labor.

Several schemes have been devised to predict gestational age from anthropometric measurements of the neonate. Table 17 compares total length and head circumference of Peruvian infants with those of London infants of known gestational age. The high altitude Cuzco infants, in respect to these measurements, fall within the range of London infants born during the fortieth week of gestation.

Data on neonatal skinfolds are difficult to interpret, since B. Gampel's study (1965) provides practically the only available comparative data. Differences in London and Lima mean skinfolds may reflect real differences in allometric growth patterns of these populations; Gampel used the left rather than the right side and the Harpenden rather than the Lange caliper, but otherwise techniques were apparently identical. In contrast to Gampel, Stanley Garn (1958), has found no reliable association between X-ray measurements of subcutaneous fat and gestational age of the neonate. The Peru-

Table 17. Comparison of infant measurements in Cuzco and Lima with those of London infants of known gestation time.

Variable	London[a]				Cuzco		Lima	
	Before term		Term					
	Boys 67	Girls 49	Boys 43	Girls 38	Boys 38	Girls 35	Boys 51	Girls 37
Birth weight (gm.)								
Mean	2,990	2,780	3,380	3,280	3,130	3,053	3,290	3,342
S.D.	550	580	370	340	458	425	477	488
Length (cm.)								
Mean	48.4	47.3	50.3	49.8	50.2	49.0	49.3	48.4
S.D.	2.5	2.9	1.9	1.5	1.6	1.4	1.9	1.1
Head circumference (cm.)								
Mean	33.6	32.5	34.6	33.7	34.5	33.8	34.1	34.2
S.D.	1.7	2.0	1.1	0.9	1.3	1.1	1.2	1.3
Triceps skinfold (mm.)								
Mean	4.5[b]	4.4	4.7	4.9	5.9	6.5	6.6	6.8
S.D.					1.5	1.7	1.0	1.3
Subscapular skinfold (mm.)								
Mean	4.5	4.8	5.0	5.4	4.4	4.3	4.4	4.7
S.D.					1.0	1.7	1.0	1.3

a From Gampel, 1965.
b Standard deviations not calculated.

vian data confirm Gampel's finding that there is no significant correlation between maternal and infant skinfolds. However, a significant correlation was found in the Lima sample between infant skinfolds and maternal parity (.05 significance: triceps, $r = .38$; .01 significance: subscapular, $r = .38$, and mean skinfold, 8 sites, $r = .38$); in the Cuzco sample only the subscapular skinfold was significantly correlated with parity (not significant: triceps, $r = .07$, and mean skinfold, 8 sites, $r = .25$; .01 significance: subscapular, $r = .39$). Gampel found no correlation between neonatal skinfolds and maternal parity.

A recent study of 300 births in Aberdeen, Scotland (Farr, 1966), reports values for skinfolds that are quite similar to those published by Gampel. Mean values for the triceps were 4.48 mm. in males and 4.84 mm. in females; means for the scapula were 4.70 mm. for males and 5.03 mm. for females. Farr notes that among term infants of normal weight females have higher mean skinfolds than do males; this relationship is reversed only among infants weighing less than 2,268 grams. Table 17 shows that the female advantage in skinfold thickness is found also in Peru; the slight male advantage in scapular skinfold in the Cuzco sample is not significant. The Aberdeen study concurred with Garn's previous study in concluding that skinfolds are a less accurate indication of gestational age than is birth weight.

There is perhaps one tentative conclusion that can be drawn from this still little understood infant variable. In malnourished infants, fatfolds are proportionately more reduced than total weight (Standard et al., 1959; Naeye, 1965b). The Cuzco data, on the other hand, show that the altitude difference in skinfolds is barely significant and not as great as the difference in birth weight (Table 12). Skinfold data thus indicate that caloric fetal malnutrition is not the mechanism depressing birth weight at high altitude.

Although total length and head circumference of the Cuzco

neonates fall within the range for full-term infants, several other indices of maturity indicate that the Cuzco population is relatively immature as compared with the Lima sample. One method of estimating infant maturity is to subtract chest circumference from head circumference; a difference of more than 2 cm. indicates possible immaturity (Usher, 1966). Using mean values for the Peruvian samples, the difference in Cuzco was greater (1.6 cm.) than was found in Lima (0.9 cm.). Another anthropometric index used to estimate maturity (Dawkins and MacGregor, 1965) is crown-rump length × 100/total length; infants with an index of 63 or less are rated immature. Inserting the sample means into this formula, an index of 64.5 was obtained for the Cuzco infants and an index of 68.0 for the Lima infants.

It is important to remember that anthropometric measurements of the day-old infant are relatively unreliable; head circumference, for example, may be more closely associated with dimensions of the mother's birth canal than with the infant's genotype or maturity. Robert Usher has pointed out in a recent article (1966) that even the more sophisticated skeletal measurements, such as X-ray examination of the tibial and femoral epiphyses, cannot distinguish immature from term infants whose growth has been retarded. Usher has proposed a set of soft-tissue criteria—development of sole creases, diameter of the breast nodule, consistency of scalp hair, and degree of ear lobe stiffening—for estimating the infant's gestational age. Application of these criteria to high altitude infants might clarify the effect of altitude on gestation time.

Of course, the ideal test would be a prospective study of high altitude pregnancy from conception to birth. The only information on gestation time available in this study was the mother's estimate, a relatively unreliable measure (Treloar et al., 1967). Seventy percent of Cuzco mothers (42/60) and 63 percent of Lima mothers (52/82) said gestation time had been normal; 22 percent of Cuzco mothers and 20 percent of Lima mothers said their pregnancy had been shorter than normal; and 8 percent of Cuzco mothers and 17 percent of Lima mothers said that length of gestation had been prolonged.

In summary, the data on infant anthropometry cannot distinguish between a slightly shortened gestation period and a slower fetal growth rate as possible mechanisms producing the birth weight depression found at high altitudes. No depression of total length or head circumference was found in the high altitude infants, in contrast to the proportional decreases reported by Lichty and his coworkers (1957) for high altitude infants in Colorado. Since no comparative data are available on normal fetal and infant growth in Peru, it is as yet impossible to interpret the altitude difference in terms of allometric growth patterns.

SURFACE AREA, UMBILICAL CORD, AND INFARCTS OF PLACENTA

Table 12 lists the differences between mean values for placental dimensions in Cuzco and Lima. The functional significance of these placental dimensions is still little understood. They do not correlate highly with any infant dimension, and Tables 18 and 19 indicate that they show few correlations among themselves.

W. Aherne and M. S. Dunnill (1966) have found that placental surface area correlates highly with placental capillary area. Their work provides the most convincing available evidence that placental area determines the capacity of the placenta to nourish and oxygenate the fetus. The highly significant negative correlation between minimum placental diameter and placental depth in the Cuzco sample (Table 19) indicates that the significant increase in diameter and the significant decrease in depth found in the Cuzco placentas may be part of a co-ordinated response of the placenta to high altitude, which increases placental area without increasing volume or weight. If the placenta is considered an ellipse, its area is equal to pi times the product of the two diameters $(A = \pi mn)$. Volume is equal to area times thickness

Table 18. Variables correlating with altitude-associated placental factors: minimum placental diameter, maximum placental depth, length of umbilical cord, and number of infarcts.

Placental factor	Correlated variable	Cuzco (11,000 ft.)		Lima (660 ft.)	
		N	r	N	r
Minimum placental diameter					
	Birth weight	73	.24[a]	88	.48[b]
	Mothers postpartum weight	60	.37[b]	75	.18
	Placental weight[c]	73	.46[b]	88	.72[b]
	Maximum placental diameter	73	.20	88	.53[b]
Maximum placental depth					
	Birth weight	73	.07	88	.22[a]
	Mother's parity	60	—.26[a]	75	—.11
	Placental weight	73	.22	88	.44[b]
	Maximum placental diameter	73	—.37[b]	88	—.13
Length of umbilical cord					
	Sex of infant[d]	73	—.29[a]	88	—.03
	Mother's postpartum weight	60	.04	75	.33[b]
	Mother's birthplace[e]	60	—.13	75	—.29[b]
Number of infarcts per placenta					
	Mother's race[f]	60	.36[b]	75	.13
	Mother's parity	60	—.29[a]	75	.23

a $P < .05$.

b $P < .01$.

c Taken by the Benirschke method, with cord and membranes cut.

d Males were coded as 1; females as 2. In Cuzco, mean cord length was 47.0 Cm. in males (N = 38; S.D. = 11.8) and 40.4 cm. in females (N = 35; S.D. = 10.0). Difference was significant ($P < .05$).

e Coded by altitude. The negative correlation means that mothers born at higher altitudes are likely to produce infants with shorter umbilical cords.

f Coded from 1 to 5, 1 being the most Indian and 5 the most European phenotype. The positive correlation means placentas of more European mothers were more likely to be infarcted in Cuzco.

Table 19. Partial coefficients of correlation between pairs of placental, maternal, and neonatal variables.

Paired variables	Held constant	Partial r	p
Minimum placental diameter Birth weight	Placental weight	.10[a]	—
Minimum placental diameter Mother's weight	Birth weight	.24[a]	.06
Minimum placental diameter Maximum placental diameter	Placental weight	.10[a]	—
Maximum placental diameter Placental depth	Placental weight	—.47[a]	.01
Umbilical cord length Mother's weight	Mother's birthplace (alt.)	.35[b]	.01
Umbilical cord length Mother's birthplace (alt.)	Mother's weight	—.20[b]	—

[a] Calculated for Cuzco data only.
[b] Calculated for Lima data only.

$(V = \pi mnt)$, and since tissue density does not usually differ significantly from that of water (1.0), this is also the expression for placental weight (Spencer, 1968). This rather straightforward calculation of placental area, incidentally, may be proportional but is not identical to the "placental surface area" measured planimetrically by Aherne and Dunnill.

In accordance with the above equations, the absolute increase in measured placental area found at high altitude was not accompanied by a significant increase in absolute placental weight. Using Benirschke's method of weighing the placental body without membranes or cord, the Cuzco mean was 510.8 grams (N = 73; s.d. = 88.3); mean weight in Lima was 484.2 grams (N = 88; s.d = 107.3). Both means are slightly higher than the 454-gram mean placental weight found by Shirley Driscoll (personal communication) in 3,316 unselected Boston births; however, mean birth weight for the Boston births was 3,309 grams, quite close to the mean for the Lima sample. The difference may be caused in part by racial differences. According to Toshio Fujikara (personal communication), placental weight of United States Negroes (mean = 432 grams; N = 8,137) is lower than the mean for United States whites (mean = 453 grams; N = 8,279). If the reproductive advantage reported for Mongoloid women (Thomson, Chun, and Baird, 1963) involves increased maternal efficiency in nourishing the fetus, high placental weights for Mongoloids would be expected.

Another variation in high altitude placentation, not listed in Table 12, is a reportedly high incidence of placenta praevia, a condition in which the placenta develops in the lower uterine segment so that it covers or adjoins the internal os. Cuzco obstetricians diagnosed 20 (27 percent) of the 73 deliveries included in the final study sample as placenta praevia. One (1 percent) of the 88 Lima deliveries was diagnosed as placenta praevia. The Lima incidence coincides with the 0.5 percent incidence found among United States births (Driscoll, personal communication).

There are two conflicting views as to the cause of placenta praevia: that it is associated with an abnormal uterine architecture which fails to guide the implanting trophoblast to the upper uterine segments, or that it results from failure of the uterine wall to supply adequate blood supply to a properly implanted trophoblast, so that, as gestation proceeds, the placenta must spread over a larger area of attachment. Placenta praevias are reported to be thinner and larger in diameter than normal placentas. The high incidence at high altitudes in Peru, if confirmed, would support the second hypothesis.

Placenta praevias were included in the final Cuzco sample, largely because their exclusion would have seriously reduced sample size. None of the Cuzco women with placenta praevia had been diagnosed prior to delivery or had experienced the complications usually associated with placenta praevia, such as hemorrhage late in pregnancy. Placenta praevia has been associated with premature delivery as well as with increased placental area, so that inclusion of these births in the Cuzco sample might have affected mean infant dimensions as well as mean placental dimensions for the high altitude sample.

However, Table 20 shows that in the Cuzco sample the group diagnosed as placenta praevia did not differ significantly in infant or placental dimensions from the mean values for normal births. Comparison with Table 12 indicates that the high incidence of placenta praevia in Cuzco does not account for any of the other significant differences between the Cuzco and Lima population.

Mean length of the umbilical cord was 6 cm. less in the Cuzco sample than was found in Lima. Cord length, however, is a relatively unreliable dimension; the measured length depends on where the cord was cut and on how much it was stretched during delivery. However, obstetricians and midwives in both Cuzco and Lima said they cut the cord at 7.5 cm. from insertion; most personnel in both hospitals had been trained in the same school, the Lima faculty of medicine, and there is no reason to expect significant differences in obstetrical techniques in Cuzco. Further, my impression was that the Cuzco umbilical cords, relative to the Lima cords, were thin in caliber and limp with a looser spiraling of the umbilical vessels. The Cuzco pattern approaches that re-

Table 20. *Dimensions of the neonate and the placenta in normal births and births diagnosed as placenta praevia in Cuzco.*

Variable	Placenta praevia		Normal births	
	Mean	S.D.	Mean	S.D.
N	20		53[a]	
Birth weight (gm.)	3,213.2	406.6	3,050.5	470.4
Infant length (cm.)	49.7	1.3	49.6	1.7
Crown-rump length (cm.)	32.1	1.2	32.1	1.5
Thoracic circumference (cm.)	32.7	1.5	32.6	1.4
Arm length (cm.)	19.3	1.0	19.7	1.0
Mean skinfold (8 sites, mm.)	4.4	0.9	4.4	0.9
Placental weight/birth weight ratio	0.17	0.03	0.17	0.03
Placental weight[b] (gm.)	538.9	83.9	500.8	88.4
Maximum placental diameter (mm.)	18.7	2.0	18.6	2.0
Minimum placental diameter (mm.)	16.4	1.2	16.1	1.9
Placental depth (mm.)	2.3	0.5	2.2	0.4
Cord length (cm.)	42.1	9.9	44.5	11.9
Number of infarcts per placenta	0.8	1.1	1.0	1.2
Percentage placentas in sample with 1 or more infarcts	45%		57%	

[a] N for infant lengths, circumferences, and skinfolds is 48.

[b] With cord and membranes removed.

ported by P. C. Tremblay and his coworkers (1965) for the umbilical cord of infants with fetal malnutrition; it is precisely the opposite of what would have been expected if the altitude variation in cord length were caused by relatively greater stretching of the cord in Lima.

Umbilical cord morphology is still uncorrelated with placental functions or with other placental dimensions. Previous studies in England (Malpas, 1964) have reported a slight correlation ($r = .25$; $N = 538$) between cord length and total placental weight. The correlation in the Lima series ($r = .22$; $N = 88$) was significant at $P = .05$; no significant correlation between placental weight and cord length was found in the Cuzco population ($r = .05$; $N = 73$). The British study reported no significant correlations between cord length and maternal parity, age, height, weight, or blood group, or with weight or sex of the neonate. Table 18 shows that cord length correlated significantly in Lima but not in Cuzco with maternal weight, and in Cuzco but not in Lima with sex of the neonate.

Malpas cites development of the umbilical cord as an example of unconditioned blood vessel growth. He has concluded that arterial pressure at the placental end of the cord cannot be affected by length of the vessels because, barring complications such as circumvolution of the cord, infants with very long cords (100 cm. or more) are no less viable than those with shorter cords. According to Malpas, cord length is more closely related to maternal genotype than to the arteriovenous pressure gradients that develop during gestation. Driscoll (personal communication) has observed that some women consistently produce very long cords over several pregnancies. Mean cord lengths in Lima were slightly lower than those reported by C. W. Walker and B. G. Pye (1960) using the same techniques in a British sample. (England: males, 56.4 cm., $N = 87$; females, 52.1 cm., $N = 90$. Lima: males, 49.9 cm., $N = 51$; females, 49.4 cm., $N = 36$.) The negative correlation between cord length and the altitude of the mother's birthplace might be an indication that the racially more Indian mothers born at high altitudes produce shorter cords because of a difference in genotype. However, holding maternal weight constant, the partial correlation between cord length and the mother's birthplace was not significant, and there was no correlation between cord length and the mother's racial classification. Furthermore, the 18 "upper class" women studied in Cuzco—although more European (racial classification = 2.9) than either the Cuzco or Lima lower class samples—also produced relatively short umbilical cords (mean = 43.5 cm.).

Further investigation of the umbilical cord is needed to separate genetic from functional influences and to quantify the qualitative differences seen in the high altitude cord. Percy Malpas and E. M. Symonds (1966) have recently developed a method for macroscopic study of the helical vessels in the umbilicus. They hypothesize that the number of turns in the helix and the handedness of these turns are governed by genetic factors. These variables have not yet been studied in Peruvian populations.

The third area of altitude-associated placental variation is an increase at high altitude in the percentage of placentas with small infarcts, areas of coagulation necrosis resulting from localized obstruction of circulation. Although diagnosis of infarcts is highly dependent on techniques of placental examination, methods were identical in both Peruvian groups, and the Lima percentage of infarcted placentas is within the range (20–30 percent—Shirley Driscoll, personal communication; Fox, 1967) of that found in Boston. Within the lower class Cuzco sample, number of infarcts per placenta was significantly correlated with the mother's race, the more European women having more placental infarcts. As would be expected from this association, the more European upper class Cuzco women had an even higher percentage of infarcted placentas than was found in the lower class (14/18 = 78 percent of the upper class placentas had one or more infarcts).

Placental infarction leads to a reduction in effective capillary bed that may amount to a loss of one half of the exchange area which would be predicted from placental weight (Aherne and Dunnill, 1966). B. J. Van den Berg and J. Yerushalmy (1966) report that the percentage of infarcted placentas in fetuses with a slow intrauterine growth rate is three times that found in the placentas of rapidly growing fetuses (26.2 percent as compared to 8 percent). Presence of infarcts is evidently associated with real impairment of placental function, and the implication of the Cuzco data is that at high altitude such impairment is more likely in European than in Indian women. No other placental anomalies were found associated with high altitude in this sample.

A recent experiment by Liliane Delaquerriere-Richardson and Enrique Valdivia (1967) provides further evidence that placental infarction is increased at high altitudes. They exposed 66 pregnant guinea pigs to simulated altitudes of 12,800 to 15,000 feet. They found massive placental infarction associated with fetal or early neonatal death in 37 percent of the altitude-exposed animals, as opposed to 6 percent in controls. There was evidence of premature aging of the placenta at high altitude: fibrin deposition and perilobular thrombi were found in 56 percent of placentas at high altitude and only 33 percent of controls. Evidence of obstruction of decidual arteries was found in 71 percent of the high altitude animals but only 6 percent of controls. If the animals were exposed to sudden rapid ascent to a hypoxic atmosphere during pregnancy, placental infarction tended to be massive and associated with basal hematomas. Animals experiencing a more gradual exposure to high altitude tended to have microinfarcts associated with small perilobular thrombi.

The mechanism responsible for this association between infarction and high altitude is not yet clear. Hypoxia might induce spasm in the musculature of uteroplacental arterioles, and this could initiate a vascular accident that would result in ischemia and infarction. This mechanism would parallel the effect of hypoxia on pulmonary vasculature (Castillo et al., 1967). Autonomic nerves have recently been seen in the human placenta (Jacobson and Chapler, 1967), so hypoxia could act through the fetal nervous system to affect placental blood flow. Other mechanisms could also lead to infarction: hypoxia-induced focal degeneration of the syncytial lining of vessels leading to thrombosis, increased uterine blood flow leading to eddying and turbulence, or polycythemia-induced increase in blood viscosity producing disturbances of blood flow.

MATERNAL FERTILITY AND NEONATAL MORTALITY

Because of the small numbers involved and the inaccuracies inherent in the interview method, no final conclusions can be drawn from the retrospective fertility information obtained from mothers in the study sample. No significant differences in maternal fertility—as measured by total pregnancies per woman, frequency of stillbirths and abortions, or age at first pregnancy—were found between mothers in the two hospitals. It should be pointed out that more than half (50/82 = 61 percent) of the Lima women had been born at altitudes of 2,000 meters or over, and this may have obscured real differences.

The 60 Cuzco women had experienced a total of 198 livebirths, or 3.3 livebirths per woman, as compared to 3.6 livebirths per woman (295/81) in the Lima sample. Thirteen (6.1 percent) of the 213 total pregnancies described by Cuzco women and 19 (6.0 percent) of the 329 pregnancies of the Lima women had ended in spontaneous abortion. Cuzco women reported a total of two stillbirths for all previous pregnancies (.06 percent); total stillborns among the Lima pregnancies was also two (.09 percent). Average age at first pregnancy was 20.0 (S.E. = ± .5) in Cuzco and 20.5 (S.E. = ± .4) in Lima. One of the Cuzco primiparas was fifteen, one was sixteen, and two were eighteen. Baker has reported (personal communication) no first pregnancies in women under eighteen years of age in the 4,000–5,000 meter altitudes south of Cuzco. If this is a real physiological limit at these higher altitudes, it evidently does not apply to the 3,400-meter altitude in Cuzco.

Although no depression of maternal fertility at high altitude was observed in these hospital populations, the data showed a significant increase in child mortality at high altitude. Thirty-three (16.7 percent) of the 198 children liveborn to Cuzco women had died before age two; the percentage for Lima women was 12.5 percent (37/295). The difference between these percentages is highly significant (P = .01). This evidence, although only a crude measure of mortality, agrees with Mazess' finding (1966)—based on vital statistics—of significantly higher neonatal mortality in highland departments of Peru.

Within the study samples themselves, three of the 100 Cuzco infants died before leaving the hospital (birth weights: 700, 1,720, 2,750) and one of the Lima infants died (birth weight: 1,000). No information on mortality was available from hospital records in Lima, but Cuzco records showed that 27 (5.7 percent) of the 470 lower class infants born in 1965 had died before leaving the hospital. Seventeen of these 27 infants were of low birth weight; thus, 46 percent (17/37) of all low birth weight infants born in 1965 died before leaving the hospital. Of the 27 infants who died in the hospital, 21 (78 percent) were males.

Although the mortality information from hospital records, like the retrospective information about maternal fertility, is incomplete and unreliable, the data indicate that the increased neonatal mortality at high altitude is significant and is associated with very high mortality among the increased percentage of infants of low birth weight.

Findings in this study of two Peruvian samples indicate that human birth at high altitude is associated with real differences in the fetus and placenta. The high and low altitude samples did not differ significantly in maternal variables known to influence fetal development, and all evidence indicates that the pattern of fetal growth observed at high altitude reflects the influence of hypoxia.

Further studies should investigate infant maturity, placenta praevia, and cord morphology at high altitude. Demonstration of an association between high altitude hypoxia and early onset of labor, site of implantation, or cord development would contribute to the understanding of the still little-known factors that govern these processes.

Data from this and other Peruvian studies (see Tables 5 and 6) indicate that the altitude effect on birth weight is not as marked in the Andes as it is in mountain areas of the United States (see Figures 1-4). The finding in the Cuzco sample of more infarcts in placentas associated with the more European neonates indicates that Mongoloids may be more resistant than Caucasians to the effect of high altitude on the efficiency of placental exchange. This should be tested in studies of placental morphology at high altitude in the United States. Little is known about racial differences in placental morphology at sea level; data from this study indicate there may be significant differences between Mongoloids and whites in placental weight and in length of the umbilical cord.

No microscopic data were included in this analysis. Sections were collected from the Cuzco placentas but have not yet been analyzed histologically. Microscopic examination could determine whether the relative increase in placental weight at high altitude results from cell-swelling, cell hyperplasia, or increased capillarity, and whether membrane-thinning is present, such as has been reported in pressure chamber experiments with human placentas in vitro (Tominaga and Page, 1966). Future studies should also include red blood cell count and hemoglobin content of maternal and cord blood. Recent developments in placental thermography provide a safe and accurate tool for determining placental blood flow. Only studies at this level can conclusively demonstrate the mechanism of the high altitude effect on the fetus.

A recent study by a group of Peruvian physicians (Chabes et al., 1967, 1968) provides valuable new information in this area. They compared 109 spontaneous, uncomplicated, singleton deliveries in Juliaca, Peru (12,551 feet) with 100 deliveries in Lima. Planimetric measurements showed that the placentas at high altitude had an increased number of capillaries per unit area and an increased number of villi. They found a significantly higher proportion of irregularly shaped placentas at high altitude than in their sea-level sample. These "other-shaped"—that is, neither round nor oval—placentas were associated with elevated levels of cord hemoglobin; the relationship was significant at the 5 percent level. They did not report whether these placentas had a higher-than-average number of infarcts, and they obtained no information about maternal race for correlation with these placental changes. In contrast to my study, the Peruvian group reports that placental weight is decreased significantly at high altitude and that placental ratio is unchanged. They weighed the placenta after cutting the cord 1 cm. from the placental body but with membranes attached; they found mean weights of 511 grams in Juliaca and 541 grams in Lima (standard deviations for these means have not yet been published). Their results contrast with weights measured with neither cord or membranes in my own study; a mean of 511 grams was found in Cuzco (12,200 feet), and the mean found in Lima was 484 grams. Table 8 illustrates the wide range of variation found in previous studies of placental weights in Lima. Since weight of the membranes may vary greatly depending on conditions of the birth, the weighing method used in my study is inherently more accurate (Benirschke, 1961). Data on total placental weight in Denver shows an increase in placental ratio over values found at sea level in the United States (Lula Lubchenco, personal communication), and the cumulative evidence from Peru indicates that the decrease in placental weght at altitudes up to 13,000 feet is proportionately much less than the decrease in birth weight (see Table 20, Figures 1-4).

Data from larger samples are needed to test possible sex differences in the fetal response to altitude and the possibly greater vulnerability of firstborns than later-borns to the birth-weight-depressing effect of high altitude. Accurate vital statistics from a larger sample might also provide data on the specific causes of death that produce the higher neonatal mortality above 10,000 feet in Peru. Information about the mortality risk for infants of low birth weight at high altitude would help solve the problem of whether these infants are immature, growth-retarded, or genetically small. Determination of the optimum birth weight for high altitude populations—the birth weight associated with minimum neonatal mortality—would also be useful in inferring the direction of the selection pressure on birth weight at high altitude.

All available evidence indicates that the neonate at high altitude is under significantly greater mortality risk than at sea level. Neonatal mortality would be expected to be even higher in the intact peasant population than in the Cuzco hospital population. Harry Tschopik (1947) observed 150 births among Aymaran villagers in Bolivia at an altitude of 3,870 meters; he found that 14 percent of those born died before six months and 25 percent died before three years. This compares with 17 percent dying before two years in the Cuzco hospital sample at 3,411 meters of altitude. Thirty-four percent of the births chronicled by Tschopik resulted in death of the child before age thirteen, which is reproductive failure in terms of maintaining population size. Monge (1948) has interpreted many of the Andean policies of the Incas as mechanisms for increasing population growth at high altitude, but few data exist on beliefs and customs relating to birth among Quechua-speaking inhabitants of the southern Peruvian highlands. How does the excess neonatal mortality at high altitudes affect desired family size or attitudes toward child-rearing in highland cultures? This entire area has been neglected in the anthropology of Andean tribes, and existing studies have not differentiated customs in highland populations from those in lowland groups (Hilger, 1957). The impression from hospital samples observed in this study was that Cuzco mothers were more dedicated "swaddlers" and more suspicious and careful with their newborn infants than mothers in Lima, but ethnographical study of intact Quechua-speaking village populations would be necessary in order to identify cultural differences specifically related to altitude.

In summary, the cumulative evidence from this and from previous studies as well as from animal experiments at high altitude indicate that human birth weight is significantly decreased and neonatal mortality is significantly increased in the hypoxic high altitude environment. Study of the epidemiology and physiology of birth in mountain areas of the United States and in the Andes is of immediate clinical importance and may lead to increased understanding of the general causes of prematurity and fetal growth retardation. Results of this study indicate that high altitude exerts strong selective pressure on the fetal and neonatal phase of the life cycle. Further study is needed to determine how this pressure is reflected in the physiological, genetic, and cultural adaptations of highland peoples.

Appendices

Bibliography

Index

Appendix I   Forms Used in Examination of the
Placenta, Neonate, and Mother

This placental examination form is a modification of the one used in the Collaborative Study on Cerebral Palsy, Mental Retardation, and Other Neurological and Sensory Disorders of Infancy and Childhood. This study began in 1958 and is sponsored by the National Institute of Neurologic Diseases and Blindness. For definitions, illustrations, and explanation of the techniques, see Benirschke, Kurt, "Examination of the Placenta," *Obst. & Gyn.* 18:309, 1961. Dr. Shirley Driscoll of the Boston Lying-In Hospital helped me select these measures from those originally described by Benirschke. We eliminated very rare categories and the variables likely to be affected by obstetrical techniques. Since the form was designed for a specific project, it assumes a small study sample and a single observer, and it emphasizes measures of placental maturity rather than other types of pathology. It is possible to preserve cord blood samples on filter paper for amino acid analysis and also formaldehyde-fixed sections of placental villous tissue for microscopic study. Previous European and South American studies have recorded "Total Placental Weight." The measurement is included in this form for comparability, but it is much less reliable than the weight as taken in the Benirschke procedure.

PLACENTAL EXAMINATION

1. Patient's identification number_____
2. Date _____
3. Total placental weight _____gms.

4. Dimensions _____cms. (large diameter)
               _____cms. (small diameter)
               _____cms. (maximum depth)
5. Shortest distance cord-placental margin _____cms.
6. Length of cord _____cms.
7. Cord blood taken: yes_____ no_____
8. Comments—cord (color, knots, no. vessels, membranous insertion) _____
9. Insertion fetal membranes: marginal_____ circummarginate _____ circumvallate_____
10. Subchorionic fibrin: patchy_____ diffuse_____
     Grade: 0_____ 1_____ 2_____ 3_____ 4_____
11. Comments—membranes and fetal surface (color, opacity of membranes, thrombosis fetal vessels, decidual necrosis, membranous edema, cysts) _____
12. Placental weight (minus cord and membranes) _____gms.
13. Consistency maternal surface: firm_____ spongy_____
14. Calcification maternal surface: surface only_____ internal _____
     Grade: 0_____ 1_____ 2_____ 3_____ 4_____
15. Comments—maternal surface (depressed area, hemorrhage, infarcts, color, intervillous thrombosis, true cyst) _____
16. Section taken: yes_____ no_____
17. General comments (shape, multiple birth, tumor) _____

EXAMINATION OF THE NEONATE

Number _____
Name _____
Mother's name _____
Father's name _____
Place of birth _____
Date of birth _____
Age at examination _____
Sex _____

Measurements

1. Weight _____
2. Length _____

3. Sitting length _____
4. Chest circumference: inspiratory_____ expiratory_____
   Mean_____
5. Cranial circumference _____
6. Cranial circumference minus mean chest circumference _____
7. Arm length _____
8. Skinfolds (3 measurements and the mean for each skinfold)
   throat   — — — —
   forearm   — — — —
   upper arm   — — — —
   juxta-nipple   — — — —
   mid-axillary   — — — —
   back   — — — —
   waist   — — — —
   calf   — — — —

Comments

EXAMINATION OF THE MOTHER

Number _____
Date _____
Place of birth _____ altitude _____
Age _____
Address _____ duration of residence _____ prior residence
_____
Duration of this pregnancy _____ complications _____ prenatal
   care_____
Dress (braids, long skirt, jacket, shawl, hat, shoes) _____
Hair (amount, color, curliness, texture) _____
Eyes _____
Photographed: yes _____ no _____
Racial class _____
Stature _____
Weight _____
Skinfolds (3 measurements and the mean for each skinfold)
   throat   — — — —
   forearm   — — — —
   upper arm   — — — —
   juxta-nipple   — — — —

mid-axillary   __ __ __ __
back   __ __ __ __
waist   __ __ __ __
calf   __ __ __ __

Cigarette smoking: yes _____ no _____ amount _____
Coca chewing: yes _____ no _____ amount _____

Comments

FERTILITY QUESTIONNAIRE

Name _____
Number _____

Now we are going to talk about your children, about those who are alive and those who are dead, about those who live with you now and about those who have been adopted by other people. If possible, we will talk about miscarriages and about any other difficulties you have had with pregnancy.

In total, how many live children have you born? Include children from all your marriages and include children who have died.
How many of your children are alive now?
How many of your children have died?
Have you adopted any children?
Have any of your own liveborn children been adopted by other people?
What are the names of your children? Let us begin with the oldest of all.
R. (Repeat name.) Is he/she the oldest of all? (next oldest?)
Did you have any pregnancies before he/she was born?
Did you have any miscarriages before he/she was born?
Did you have any stillborns or children who later died before he/she was born?
How old is he/she now? If not now living, at what age did he/she die?
What caused his/her death?
Did he/she have a twin?
What is the name of the next child you bore?

FERTILITY HISTORY

Number of Pregnancy (note twinning)	Outcome of Pregnancy (miscarriage, stillbirth, livebirth, complications)	Sex of Child	Still Alive?	Age or Age at Death	Cause of Death

(Return to R and repeat this series of questions until all children have been listed.)

How old were you when you had your first pregnancy?

SOCIAL HISTORY OF MOTHER

What is the first language that you learned to speak? Quechua _____ Aymara _____ Spanish _____

Can you read this language? Write it? Both read and write?

What other languages do you speak now? Quechua _____ Aymara _____ Spanish _____

Can you read or write this second language?

Do you speak Spanish? None_____ A few words_____ Fluently _____

Did you go to school? How many years?

Are you working now?

What kind of work?

Appendix II   List of Variables Coded for Statistical Analysis

For each case there are four cards:
   Card 1—Placental dimensions and pathology
   Card 2—Anthropometry of the newborn
   Card 3—Anthropometry of the mother; race
   Card 4—Maternal fertilty
Columns 1-36 are identical for all four cards. The core information contains (a) identification, (b) rejection criteria, and (c) data that should be correlated with information on all cards.

CORE INFORMATION

Column	Variable	No. columns
1-3	Number: 0–100-Cuzco; 101–200-Lima	3
4	Place: 1-Cuzco; 2-Lima	1
5	Sex: 1-male; 2-female	1
6-9	Birthweight: ex. 2450 gm.	4
10	Abnormalities of newborn: 1-absent; 2-present; 3-multiple; 4-infant nonviable	1
11-12	Type of abnormality: 1-stillborn; 2-incubator; 3-died first 20 days; 4-cyanotic; 5-other. (If applicable, use 2 code numbers.)	1 & 1
13	Economic status: 1-ward; 2-private	1
14	Infant birthweight class: 1-< 500 gm.; 2-<1000; 3-<1500; 4-<2000; 5-<2500; 6-<3000; 7-<3500; 8-<4000, 9-<4500	1

115

Column	Variable	No. columns
15	Gestational age (mother's estimate): 1-normal; 2-less than normal; 3-longer than normal	1
16	Race (observer's assessment of mother): 1, 2, 3, 4, 5 = gradations Quechua to Spanish; 6-Negroid; 7-Chinese	1
17-18	Mother's age: ex. 28 yr.	2
19-21	Mother's weight: ex. 50.5 kg.	3
22-23	Number of pregnancy: ex. 09	2
24-25	Number of birth: ex. 07	2
26	Abnormality of pregnancy: 1-absent; 2-present; 3-multiple	1
27-28	Type: 1-pre-eclampsia: 2-toxemia; 3-anemia; 4-bleeding; 5-other	1 & 1
29	Abnormality of delivery: 1-absent; 2-present; 3-multiple	1
30-31	Type: 1-Caesarean section; 2-placenta praevia; 3-placental retention; 4-hemorrhage; 5-twin birth; 6-breech birth; 7-cord complication; 8-other	1 & 1
32	Card 2 complete: 1-yes; 2-no	1
33	Card 3 complete: 1-yes; 2-no; 3-partial (no ht. & wt.)	1
34-36	Placental ratio (Benirschke): ex. .192	3

CARD 1—PLACENTA

Column	Variable	No. columns
1-36	Core information	36
37-40	Placental weight (total): ex. 0630 gm., 1200 gm.	4
41-43	Placental weight (Benirschke): ex. 520 gm.	3
44-46	Maximum diameter: ex. 17.1 cm.	3
47-49	Minimum diameter: ex. 14.0 cm.	3
50-51	Maximum depth: ex. 2.5 cm.	2
52-54	Cord length: ex. 30.1 cm.	3

Column	Variable	No. columns
55-56	Distance cord insertion-margin: ex. 3.5 cm.	2
57	Cord insertion: 1-normal; 2-marginal; 3-membranous	1
58	Subchorionic fibrin (grade): 1-absent; 2-grade 1; 3-grade 2; 4-grade 3; 5-grade 4	1
59	Fibrin distribution: 1-absent; 2-diffuse; 3-patchy; 4-both patchy and diffuse	1
60	Calcification maternal surface: graded as for fibrin 1-5	1
61	Calcification distribution; 1-surface only; 2-internal; 3-absent	1
62	Number of infarcts: ex. 0	1
63	Meconium: 1-absent; 2-present	1
64	Abnormalities maternal surface: 1-absent; 2-present; 3-multiple	1
65	Abnormalities cord, fetal surface, membranes; 1-absent; 2-present; 3-multiple	1
66-68	Placental ratio (total): ex. .194	3
69-71	Infant stature: ex. 49.8 cm.	3
72-73	Abnormalities maternal surface (type): 1-depressed area; 2-thrombosis; 3-extra lobe; 4-other; 9-incomplete	1 & 1
74-75	Abnormalities fetal surface, cord, membranes (type): 1-membrane insertion; 2-decidual necrosis, membranes; 3-cord abnormalities; 4-color; 5-cyst; 6-membrane abnormalities; 7-other	1 & 1
76	Placental discard: blank—include all data; 2-discard: immature, giant, twins; 3-discard: caesarean, ? completeness	1
77-78	Blank	2
79	Total abnormalities (72–73 & 74–75 & infarcts): 1-none; 2-one; 3-two; 4-three or more	1
80	Card number: 1	1

CARD 2: NEWBORN

Column	Variable	No. columns
1-36	Core material	36
37-39	Stature: ex. 49.5 cm.	3
40-42	Crown-rump length: ex 33.2 cm.	3
43-45	Cranial circumference: ex. 32.0 cm.	3
46-48	Thoracic circumference: ex. 31.0 cm.	3
49-51	Arm length: ex. 21.5 cm.	3
	Skinfolds (ex. 12 mm., 05 mm.)	
52-53	Chin	2
54-55	Forearm	2
56-57	Triceps	2
58-59	Breast 1	2
60-61	Breast 2	2
62-63	Subscapular	2
64-65	Waist	2
66-67	Leg	2
68-69	Total	2
70-71	Mean: ex. 3.1 mm.	2
72-73	Thoracic circumference/height (ratio): ex. .75	2
74-75	Blank	2
76	Cranial minus thoracic circumference: 1-positive value; 2-negative value	1
77-78	Cranial minus thoracic circumference: ex. 1.5 cm.	2
79	Blank	1
80	Card number: 2	1

CARD 3: MOTHER

Column	Variable	No. columns
1-36	Core material	36
37-40	Mother's stature: ex 143.2 cm.	4
41	Quechua: 1-first language; 2-second language; 3-not fluent; 4-no knowledge	1
42	Spanish: 1–4, as for Quechua	1

Column	Variable	No. columns
43-44	Years of school: 00–12	2
45-46	Years of residence: 00–45	2
47	Birthplace (altitude): 1-0–1000 meters; 2-1001–2000; 3-2001–2500; 4-2501–3000; 5-3001–3500; 6-3501 & over	1
48	Paid work: 1-none; 2-light; 3-heavy	1
	Skinfolds (ex. 20 mm., 09 mm) ;	
49-50	Chin	2
51-52	Forearm	2
53-54	Triceps	2
55-56	Breast 1	2
57-58	Breast 2	2
59-60	Subscapular	2
61-62	Waist	2
63-64	Leg	2
65-67	Total: ex. 090 mm.	3
68-70	Mean: ex. 14.9 mm.	3
71	Birthplace: 1-Cuzco; 2-Lima; blank-others	1
72	Resident class: 1-less than one year; 2-one to five years; 3-six to ten years; 4-eleven years or more	1
73-79	Blank	6
80	Card number: 3	1

CARD 4: FERTILITY

Column	Variable	No. columns
1-36	Core material	36
37	Total boys liveborn	1
38	Total girls liveborn	1
39	Total pregnancies: 1-1; 2-2; 3-3 or 4; 4-5 or more	1
40	Blank	1
41	Total boys living	1
42	Total girls living	1
43	Boys who died age 0-1 year	1
44	Boys who died age 1-3 years	1

Column	*Variable*	*No. columns*
45	Boys who died age 3 years and older	1
46	Total boys dead	1
47	Girls who died age 0-1 year	1
48	Girls who died age 1-3 years	1
49	Girls who died age 3 years and older	1
50	Total girls dead	1
51	Total children dead	1
52-53	Age first pregnancy	2
54-56	Interval (months) since last pregnancy	3
57	Number of abortions	1
58	Number of stillbirths	1
59-73	Pregrancy 1 to n; 1-normal birth; 2-abortion; 3-stillbirth; 4-child who died: 5-twinbirth; 6-caesarean; 8-immature child	14 (each treated as a separate variable
74-76	Liveborn boys/liveborn girls	3
77-78	Blank	2
79	Outcome last prior pregnancy: 1-normal birth; 2-abortion; 3-stillbirth; 4-child who died; 5-twinbirth; 6-caesarean; 7-first pregnancy coded; none prior; 8-immature child; 9-no fertility information	1
80	Card number: 4	1

Bibliography

Aberle, S. B. D. 1930. "The Relation of the Weight of the Placenta, Cord, and Membranes to the Weight of the Infant in Normal Full-Term and in Premature Deliveries." *Am. J. Obstet. Gynec.*, 20: 397-404.

Abernathy, J. R., B. G. Greenberg, J. E. Grizzle, and J. F. Donnelly. 1966. "Birth Weight, Gestation, and Crown-Heel Length as Response Variables in Multivariate Analysis." *Am. J. Public Health*, 56:1281-1286.

Abramowicz, Mark, and E. H. K. Kass. 1966. "Pathogenesis and Prognosis of Prematurity." *New Eng. J. Med.*, 275: 878-885, 938-943, 1001-1007.

Acosta Chavez, M. H. 1964. "Algunos Aspectos del Nino Primaturo en las Alturas; Estudio Clinico-Estadistico Realizado en el Hospital de Huaron a 4,750 Metros de Altura Sobre el Nivel del Mar." Thesis 5886, Facultad de Medicina, Lima.

Acurio, Romulo. 1965. "Somatometria del Recien Nacido en la Altura." Unpublished Ms., Cuzco.

Adair, F. L., and Hulda Thelander. 1925. "A Study of the Weight and Dimensions of the Human Placenta in Its Relation to the Weight of the Newborn Infant." *Am. J. Ostet. Gynec.*, 10:172-205.

Aherne, W. 1966. "A Weight Relationship Between the Human Fetus and Placenta." *Biol. Neonat.*, 10: 113-118.

Aherne. W., and M. S. Dunnill. 1966. "Morphometry of the Human Placenta." *Brit. Med. Bull.*, 22: 5-8.

Altland, P. D. 1949. "Breeding Performance of Rats Exposed Repeatedly to 18,000 Feet." *Physiol. Zool.*, 22: 232-246.

Altland, P. D., and Benjamin Highman. 1964. "Effects of Age and Exercise on Altitude Tolerance in Rats," in W. H. Weihe, ed. *The Physiological Effects of High Altitude.* New York: Pergamon Press.

Altland, P. D., and Benjamin Highman. 1968. "Sex Organ Changes and Breeding Performance of Male Rats Exposed to Altitude: Effect of Exercise and Physical Training." *J. Reprod. Fert.*, 15: 215-222.

Alzamora, Orlando. 1958. "Algunas Observaciones Sobre Alteraciones de la Placenta en la Altura." *Rev. Assoc. Med. Yauli*, III; 75-81.

Alzamora-Castro, V. 1952. "Sobre la Posible Influencia de las Grandes Alturas en la Determinacion de Algunas Malformaciones Cardiacas." *Rev. Peru. Cardiol.* (Lima), 1: 189-198.

Anderson, Henning. 1966. "The Influence of Hormones on Human Development," in Frank Falkner, ed. *Human Development*. Philadelphia: W. B. Saunders.

Anderson, Mavis, L. N. Went, J. E. MacIver, and H. G. Dixon. 1960. "Sickle-Cell Disease in Pregnancy." *Lancet*, 2: 516-521.

Arias-Stella, Javier, and Yolanda Castillo. 1966. "The Muscular Pulmonary Arterial Branches in Stillborn Natives of High Altitude." *Lab. Invest.*, 15: 1951-1959.

Arias-Stella, Javier, and Hever Kruger. 1963. "Pathology of High Altitude Pulmonary Edema." *Arch. Path.*, 76: 147-157.

Armitage, P., J. D. Boyd, W. J. Hamilton, and B. C. Rowe, 1967. "A Statistical Analysis of a Series of Birthweights and Placental Weights." *Hum. Biol.*, 39: 430-444.

Assali, N. S. 1967. "Some Aspects of Fetal Life in Utero and the Changes at Birth." *Am. J. Obstet. Gynec.*, 97: 324-331.

Babson, S. G., and C. M. McKinnon. 1968. "Determination of Gestational Age in Premature Infants." *Lancet*, 1: 174-177.

Baird, Sir Dugald. 1964. "The Epidemiology of Prematurity." *J. Pediat.*, 65: 909-924.

Baker, P. T. 1959. "American Negro-White Differences in the Thermal Insulative Aspects of Body Fat." *Hum. Biol.*, 31: 316-323.

Baker, P. T. 1966. "Ecological and Physiological Adaptation in Indigenous South Americans: With Special Reference to the Physical Environment," in P. T. Baker and J. S. Weiner, eds. *The Biology of Human Adaptability*. Oxford: Clarendon Press.

Baker, P. T., E. R. Buskirk, J. Kollias, and R. B. Mazess. 1967. "Temperature Regulation at High Altitude: Quechua Indians and U.S. Whites During Total Body Cold Exposure." *Hum. Biol.*, 39: 155-169.

Baker, P. T., A. R. Frisancho, M. A. Little, R. B. Mazess, and R. B. Thomas. 1965. *A Preliminary Study of the Cultural and Biological*

Characteristics of a Peruvian Highland Population: Annual Progress Report. The Pennsylvania State University: University Park, Pennsylvania.

Baker, P. T., E. E. Hunt, Jr., and Tulkia Sen. 1958. "The Growth and Interrelations of Skinfolds and Brachial Tissues in Man." *Am. J. Phys. Anthrop.,* 16: 39-58.

Bakwin, Harrry. 1964. "The Secular Change in Growth and Development." *Acta. Paediat. Scand.,* 53: 79-89.

Barbashova, Z. I. 1964. "Cellular Level of Adaptation," in D. B. Dill, E. F. Adolf, and C. B. Wilber, eds. *Handbook of Physiology.* Washington, D. C.: American Physiological Society.

Barker, J. N. 1957. "Role of Hemoglobin Affinity and Concentration in Determining Hypoxia Tolerance of Mammals During Infancy, Hypoxia, and Irradiation." *Am. J. Physiol.,* 189: 281-289.

Barron, D. H., James Metcalfe, Giacomo Meschia, Andre Hellegers, Harry Prystowsky, and William Huckabee. 1964. "Adaptations of Pregnant Ewes and Their Fetuses to High Altitude," in W. H. Weihe, ed. *The Physiological Effects of High Altitude.* New York: Pergamon Press.

Battaglia, F. C., and L. O. Lubchenco. 1967. "A Practical Classification of Newborn Infants by Weight and Gestational Age." *J. Pediat.,* 71: 159-163.

Benirschke, Kurt. 1961. "Examination of the Placenta." *Obstet. Gynec.,* 18: 309-333.

Benirschke, Kurt. 1965. "Major Pathologic Features of the Placenta, Cord, and Membranes," in *Symposium on the Placenta: Its Form and Function with Reference to the Prevention of Birth Defects and Fetal Deaths.* New York: National Foundation March of Dimes.

Bennett, C. G., and L. S. Louis. 1959. "Demographic Factors Influencing Birth Weight." *Hawaii M. J.,* 18: 239-244.

Berensohn, S., and M. Muro. 1957. "Constantes Hematologicas en Mujeres Residentes en las Grandes Alturas." *An. Fac. Med.* (Lima), 40: 925-935.

Bresler, J. B. 1962. "Maternal Height and the Prevalance of Stillbirths." *Am. J. Phys. Anthrop.,* 20: 515-517.

Brimblecombe, F. S. W., J. R. Ashford, and J. G. Fryer. 1968. "Significance of Low Birth Weight in Perinatal Mortality." *Brit. J. Prev. Soc. Med.,* 22: 27-35.

Bromberg, Y. M., H. S. Halevi, and A. Brzezinsky. 1951. "Studies in

Anthropometry of Jewish Infants in Palestine." *Am. J. Phys. Anthrop.*, 9: 297-310.

Calderon, Rolando, Alberto Uerena, Leopoldo Munive, and Francisco Kruger. 1966. "Intravenous Glucose Tolerance Test in Pregnancy in Women Living in Chronic Hypoxia." *Diabetes,* 15: 130-132.

Campos Rey De Castro, Jorge and B. Iglesias. 1956. "Mechanisms of Natural Acclimatization: Preliminary Report on Anatomic Studies at High Altitudes." Randolph AFB, Texas: USAF School of Aviation Medicine.

Castillo, Y., H. Kruger, J. Arias-Stella, A. Hurtado, P. Harris, and D. Heath. 1967. "Histology, Extensability, and Chemical Composition of Pulmonary Trunk in Persons Living at Sea-Level and at High Altitude in Peru." *Brit. Heart J.*, 29: 120-128.

Cawley, R. H., Thomas McKeown, and R. G. Record. 1954. "Parental Stature and Birth Weight." *Am. J. Hum. Gen.*, 6: 448-456.

Chabes, A., J. Pereda, J. Perez, N. Barrientos, A. Monroe, and L. Campos. 1967. "Morphometry of Human Placenta at High Altitude, Abstracted." *Am. J. Path.*, 50: 14a-15a.

Chabes, Alvaro, Jose Pereda, Lyon Hyams, Nicolas Barrientos, Jaime Perez, Luis Campos, Adolfo Monroe, and Americo Mayorga. 1968. "Comparative Morphometry of the Human Placenta at High Altitude and at Sea Level: The Shape of the Placenta." *Obstet. Gynec.*, 31: 178-185.

Chiodi, Hugo. 1964. "Action of High Altitude Chronic Hypoxia on Newborn Animals," in W. H. Weihe, ed. *The Physiological Effects of High Altitude.* New York: Pergamon Press.

Clavero-Nunez, J. A., and J. Botella-Lluria. 1963. "Ergebnisse von Messungen der Gesamtoberflache Normaler und Krankhafter Placenten." *Arch. Gynaek.*, 198: 56-60.

Connor, Angie, C. G. Bennett, and L. S. K. Louis. 1957. "Birth Weight Patterns by Race in Hawaii." *Hawaii M. J.*, 16: 626-632.

Cook, S. F., and A. A. Krum. 1955. "Determination of Mouse Strains Exposed for Long Periods to Low Atmospheric Pressure." *J. Exp. Zool.*, 128: 561-572.

Cotter, J. R., J. N. Blechner, and Harry Prystowsky. 1967. "Observations on Pregnancy at High Altitude: The Respiratory Gases in Maternal Arterial and Uterine Venous Blood." *Am. J. Obstet. Gynec.*, 99: 1-8.

Cruz-Jibaya, Julio, Natalio Banchero, Francisco Sime, Dante Penaloza, Raul Gamboa, and Emilio Marticorena. 1964. "Correlation Between Pulmonary Arterial Pressure and Level of Altitude." *Dis. Chest*, 46: 446-451.

Cuellas Huapaya, F. R. 1962. "Estudio Morfologico de Placentas Procedientes de Gestaciones Normales y Patologicas." Thesis 5439, Facultad de Medicina, Lima.

Damon, Albert. 1966. "Negro-White Differences in Pulmonary Function." *Hum. Biol.*, 38: 380-393.

Dancis, Joseph. 1959. "The Placenta." *J. Pediat.*, 55: 85-101.

Dancis, Joseph. 1965. "The Role of the Placenta in Fetal Survival." *Ped. Clin. N. Amer.*, 12: 1-9.

Davis, Kingsley, and Judith Blake. 1956. "Social Structure and Fertility." *Econ. Dev. and Cultural Change*, 4: 211-235.

Dawes, G. S. 1961. "Oxygen Consumption and Hypoxia in the Newborn Animal," in G. W. Wolstenholme and Maeve O'Connor, eds. *Ciba Foundation Symposium on Somatic Stability in the Newly Born*. Boston: Little, Brown and Company.

Dawkins, Michael, and W. G. MacGregor, eds. 1965. *Gestational Age, Size and Maturity. A Symposium*. London: Spastics Society Medical Education and Information Unit.

Debias, D. A. 1966. "Thyroid-Adrenal Relationship in Altitude Tolerance." *Fed. Proc.* 25: 1227-1232.

Delaquerriere-Richardson, Liliane, and Enrique Valdivia. 1967. "Effects of Simulated High Altitude on Pregnancy: Placental Morphology in Albino Guinea Pigs." *Arch. Path.*, 84: 405-417.

Driscoll, S. G. 1965. "The Pathology of Pregnancy Complicated by Diabetes Mellitus." *Med. Clin. N. Amer.*, 49: 1053-1065.

Duda Vegas, Ronald. 1962. "Talla y Peso del Recien Nacido en Huancayo." *Rev. Assoc. Med. Yauli*, VII: 83-95.

Ellis, R. W. B., and D. N. Lavley. 1951. "Assessment of Prematurity by Birth Weight, Crown-Rump Length and Head Circumference." *Arch. Dis. Child.*, 26: 411-422.

Ely, B. 1962. "Etude d'un Groupe de Tsiganes au Point de Vue Obstetrical." *Bulletins et Memoires de la Societe d'Anthropologie de Paris*, 3: 224-228.

Erhardt, C. L., G. B. Joshi, F. G. Nelson, B. H. Kroll, and Louis Weiner. 1964. "Influence of Weight and Gestation on Perinatal Mortality by Ethnic Group." *Am. J. Public Health*, 54: 1841-1855.

Falkner, Frank. 1966. "General Considerations in Human Development," in Frank Falkner, ed. *Human Development*. Philadelphia: W. B. Saunders.

Farr, Valerie. 1966. "Skinfold Thickness as an Indication of Maturity of the Newborn." *Arch. Dis. Child.*, 41: 301-308.

Feigen, G. A., and P. K. Johnson. 1962. "Blood Volumes and Heart Weights in Two Strains of Rats During Adaptation to a Natural Altitude of 12,470 Feet," in W. H. Weihe, ed. *The Physiological Effects of High Altitude.* New York: Pergamon Press.

Folk, G. E. 1966. *Introduction to Environmental Physiology: Environmental Extremes and Mammalian Survival.* Philadelphia: Lea and Febiger.

Fox, H. 1967. "The Significance of Placental Infarction in Perinatal Morbidity and Mortality." *Biol. Neonat.*, 11: 87-105.

Fraccaro, Marco. 1956. "A Contribution to the Study of Birth Weight Based on an Italian Sample." *Ann. Hum. Gen.*, 20: 282-298.

Gampel, B. 1965. "The Relation of Skinfold Thickness in the Neonate to Sex, Length of Gestation, Size at Birth and Maternal Skinfold." *Hum. Biol.*, 37: 29-37.

Garn, S. M. 1958. "Fat, Body Size and Growth in the Newborn." *Hum. Biol.*, 30: 265-280.

Garn, S. M., and Zui Shamir. 1958. *Methods for Research in Human Growth.* Springfield, Illinois: Charles Thomas.

Gomero Espiritu, Raul. 1965. "Volumen Cardiaco en Gestantes de la Altura y su Relacion con el Peso del Recien Nacido." Thesis 6140, Facultad de Medicina, Lima.

Grabowski, C. T. 1964. "The Etiology of Hypoxia-Induced Malformations in the Chick Embryo." *J. Exp. Zool.*, 157: 307-325.

Grahn, Douglas, and Jack Kratchman. 1963. "Variation in Neonatal Death Rate and Birth Weight in the United States and Possible Relations to Environmental Radiation, Geology and Altitude." *Am. J. Hum. Genet.*, 15: 329-352.

Griswold, D. M., and Denis Cavanagh. 1966. "Prematurity—the Epidemiologic Profile of the 'High Risk' Mother." *Am. J. Obstet. Gynec.*, 96: 878-882.

Gruenwald, Paul, and H. N. Minh. 1961. "Evaluation of Body and Organ Weights in Perinatal Pathology: Weight of Body and Placenta in Surviving and of Autopsied Infants." *Am. J. Obstet. Gynec.*, 82: 312-319.

Gruenwald, Peter. 1963. "Chronic Fetal Distress and Placental Insufficiency." *Biol. Neonat.*, 5: 215-223.

Gruenwald, Peter. 1966. "Growth of the Human Fetus: Normal

Growth and Its Variation." *Am. J. Obstet. Gynec.*, 94: 1112-1132.

Gruenwald, Peter, Hatao Funakawa, Sigeru Mitani, Toshio Nishimura, and Shigaki Takeuchi. 1967. "Influence of Environmental Factors on Foetal Growth in Man." *Lancet*, 1: 1026-1028.

Hafez, E. S. E. 1963. "Maternal Influence on Fetal Size." *Int. J. Fertil.*, 8: 547-553.

Hafez, E. S. E. 1967. "Reproductive Failure in Domestic Mammals," in Kurt Benirschke, ed. *Comparative Aspects of Reproductive Failure.* New York: Springer-Verlag.

Harper, P. A., and G. Wiener. 1965. "Sequelae of Low Birth Weight." *Ann. Rev. Med.* 16: 405-420.

Harris, C. W., J. L. Shields, and J. P. Hannon. 1966. "Acute Altitude Sickness in Females." *Aerospace Med.*, 37: 1163-1167.

Harris, C. W., J. L. Shields, and J. P. Hannon. 1966. "Electrocardiographic and Radiographic Heart Changes in Women at High Altitude." *Am. J. Cardiol.*, 18: 847-854.

Harrison, G. A. 1966. "Human Adaptability with Reference to the IBP Proposals for High-Altitude Research," in P. T. Baker and J. S. Weiner, eds. *The Biology of Human Adaptability.* Oxford: Clarendon Press.

Harrison, G. A., and J. S. Weiner. 1964. "Human Evolution," in J. S. Weiner, J. M. Tanner, and N. A. Barnicot, eds. *Human Biology.* New York: Oxford University Press.

Haworth, J. C., Louise Dilling, and M. K. Younoszai. 1967. "Relation of Blood-Glucose to Haematocrit, Birthweight and Other Body Measurements in Normal and Growth-Retarded Newborn Infants." *Lancet*, 2: 901-905.

Hellegers, Andre, James Metcalfe, W. E. Huckabee, Harry Prystowsky, Giacomo Meschia, and D. H. Barron, 1961. "Alveolar PCO2 and PO2 in Pregnant and Non-Pregnant Women at High Altitude." *Am. J. Obstet. Gynec.*, 82: 241-245.

Hellriegel, K. O. 1963. "El Ductus Arterioso Persistente: Observaciones Hechas en las Grandes Alturas." *Rev. Asoc. Med. Yauli*, VIII: 20-31.

Hendricks, C. H. 1964. "Patterns of Fetal and Placental Growth: The Second Half of Normal Pregnancy." *Obstet. Gynec.*, 24: 357-365.

Hendricks, C. H. 1967. "Delivery Patterns and Reproductive Efficiency Among Groups of Differing Socioeconomic Status and Ethnic Origins." *Am. J. Obstet. Gynec.*, 97: 608-624.

Hewitt, David. 1963. "Further Observations on Seasonal Parturition." *Am. J. Obstet. Gynec.*, 85: 695-697.

Hewitt, David, and Alice Stewart. 1952. "The Oxford Child Health Survey: A Study of the Influence of Social and Genetic Factors on Infant Weight." *Hum. Biol.*, 24: 309-319.

Hilger, M. I. 1957. *Araucanian Child Life and Its Cultural Background.* Washington D.C.: Smithsonian Institute.

Hobbs, J. R., and J. A. Davis. 1967. "Serum Gamma G-Globulin Levels and Gestational Age in Premature Babies." *Lancet*, 1: 757-759.

Hollingsworth, M. J. 1965. "Observations on the Birth Weights and Survival of African Babies: Single Births." *Ann. Hum. Genet.*, 28: 291-300.

Hollingsworth, M. J., and Catherine Duncan. 1966. "The Birth Weight and Survival of Ghanaian Twins." *Ann. Hum. Genet.*, 30: 13-24.

Hosemann, Hans. 1949. "Schwangerschaftsdauer und Gewicht der Placenta." *Arch. Gynakol.*, 176: 453-457.

Hosemann, Hans. 1950. "Kindliche Masse und Neugeborenensterblichkeit." *Naturwissenschaften*, 37: 409-415.

Houghton, J. W., and W. F. Ross. 1953. "Birth Weights and Prematurity in Southern Rhodesia." *Trans. Roy. Soc. Trop. Med. Hyg.*, 47: 62-65.

Hueneman, R. L. 1954. "Nutrition and Care of Young Children in Peru." *J. Am. Diet. Ass.*, 30: 554-569, 1101-1109; 31: 1121-1133.

Hunt, E. E. 1966. "The Developmental Genetics of Man," in Frank Falkner, ed. *Human Development.* Philadelphia: W. B. Saunders.

Hurtado, Alberto. 1955. "Hombre y Ambiente: El Hombre en las Grandes Alturas Habitadas." *An. Fac. Med. Lima*, 33: 9-16.

Hurtado, Alberto. 1956. "Aspectos Patologicos de la Vida en las Grandes Alturas." *An. Fac. Med. Lima*, 39: 957-976.

Hurtado, Alberto. 1960. "Some Clinical Aspects of Life at High Altitudes." *Ann. Int. Med.*, 53: 247-258.

Hurtado, Alberto. 1962. *The Physiological Effects of High Altitude.* New York: Pergamon Press.

Hurtado, Alberto. 1964. "Animals in High Altitudes: Resident Man," in D. B. Dill, E. F. Adolf, and C. B. Wilber, eds. *Handbook of Physiology.* Washington, D. C.: American Physiological Society.

Ichaliotis, S. D., and T. C. Lambrinopoulos. 1964. "Les Correlations Entre le Poids du Placenta et le Taux de l'Oxytocinase du Serum." *Gynec. Obstet.* (Paris), 63: 543-548.

Ingalls, T. H., and F. J. Curley. 1957. "Principles Governing the

Genesis of Congenital Malformations Induced in Mice by Hypoxia." *New Eng. J. Med.* 257: 1121-1127.

Ingalls, T. H., F. J. Curley, and R. A. Prindle. 1952. "Experimental Production of Congenital Anomalies." *New Eng. J. Med.*, 247: 758-768.

Interdepartmental Committee on Nutrition for National Defense (ICNND). 1959. "Nutrition Survey of the Armed Forces, Peru." Washington, D. C.

Jacobsen, H. N., and F. K. Chapler. 1967. "Intrinsic Innervation of the Human Placenta." *Nature*, 214: 103-104.

James, L. S., and E. D. Burnard. 1961. "Biochemical Changes Occurring During Asphyxia and Some Effects on the Heart," in G. W. Wolstenholme and Maeve O'Connor, eds. *Ciba Foundation Symposium on Somatic Stability in the Newly Born.* Boston: Little, Brown and Company.

Jara Velarde, J. A. 1961. "Evaluacion y Somatometria del Recien Nacido, Estudio Comparativo en La Oroya y Lima." Thesis 5194, Facultad de Medicina, Lima.

Jayant, R. 1964. "Birth Weight and Some Other Factors in Relation to Infant Survival: A Study on an Indian Sample." *Ann. Hum. Gen.*, 27: 261-270.

Jelliffe, E. F. 1966. "Malaria Infection of the Placenta and Low Birth Weight (A Preliminary Communication)." *J. Trop. Pediat.*, 12: 15.

Johnson, Duane, and P. G. Roofe. 1965. "Blood Constituents of Normal Newborn Rats and Those Exposed to Low Oxygen Tension During Gestation; Weight of Newborn and Litter Size Also Considered." *Anat. Rec.*, 153: 303-309.

Kaiser, I. H., J. N. Cummings, S. R. M. Reynolds, and J. P. Marbarger. 1958. "Acclimatization Response of the Pregnant Ewe and Fetal Lamb to Diminished Ambient Pressure." *J. Appl. Physiol.*, 13: 171-178.

Kang, Yung Sun. 1962. "Sex Ratio and Other Attributes of the Neonate in Korea." *Hum. Biol.*, 34: 38-48.

Karn, M. N., and L. S. Penrose. 1951. "Birth Weight and Gestation Time in Relation to Maternal Age, Parity and Infant Survival." *Ann. Eugenics*, 16: 147-164.

Kerpel-Fronius, E., F. Varga, and G. Mestyan. 1961. "Clinical Aspects of Stability," in G. W. Wolstenholme and Maeve O'Connor, eds. *Ciba Foundation Symposium on Somatic Stability in the Newly Born.* Boston: Little, Brown and Company.

Keys, Ansel. 1935. "The Physiology of Life at High Altitude: Paper of the International High Altitude Expedition to Chile." *The Scientific Monthly*, 63: 289-312.

Keys, Ansel, Ernst Simonson, A. S. Skinner, and S. M. Wells. 1950. "Growth and Development," in A. Keys et al., eds. *The Biology of Human Starvation*, Vol. II. Minneapolis: The University of Minnesota Press.

Khoury, G. H., and C. R. Hawes. 1967. "Atrial Septal Defect Associated with Pulmonary Hypertension in Children Living at High Altitude." *J. Pediat.*, 70: 432-435.

Knox, George, and David Morley. 1960. "Twinning in Yoruba Women." *J. Obstet. Gynaec. Brit. Emp.*, 67: 981-984.

Koskela, Osmo. 1965. "Large Fetus: A Geographic Modification." *Ann. Chir. Gynaec. Fenn.*, 54: 462-471.

Kouvalainen, Kauko, and Kalle Osterlund. 1967. "Placental Weights in Down's Syndrome." *Ann. Med. Exp. Fenn.*, 45: 320-322.

Kreuzer, F. 1967. "Transport of Oxygen and Carbon Dioxide at Altitude," in Rodolfo Margaria, ed. *Exercise at Altitude*. Amsterdam: Excerpta Medica Foundation.

Latham, M. C., and J. R. K. Robson. 1966. "Birthweight and Prematurity in Tanzania." *Trans. Roy. Soc. Trop. Med. Hyg.*, 60: 791-796.

Leitch, J. A. 1961. "Incidence and Effects of Prematurity Among Non-Africans in Ndola, Northern Rhodesia." *Cent. Afn. J. Med.*, 7: 279-284.

Levine, Bernard, C. W. Ely, and W. A. Wood. 1966. "Assessment of Fetal Maturity by Maternal Serum Alkaline Phosphatase Analysis." *Am. J. Obstet. Gynec.*, 96: 1155-1158.

Lichty, J. A., R. Y. Ting, P. D. Bruns, and Elizabeth Dyar. 1957. "Studies of Babies Born at High Altitudes: I. Relation of Altitude to Birth Weight. II. Measurement of Birth Weight, Body Length, and Head Size. III. Arterial Oxygen Saturation and Hematocrit Values at Birth." *Am. Med. Assoc. Dis. Child.*, 93: 666-677.

Loewy, Adolf, and Eric Wittkower. 1937. *The Pathology of High Altitude Climate, With Contributions to the Climatology of Highland Regions and to the Constitution of Highland Inhabitants.* London: Oxford University Press.

Love, E. J., and R. A. H. Kinch. 1965 "Factors Influencing the Birth Weight in Normal Pregnancy." *Am. J. Obstet. Gynec.*, 91: 342-349.

McDonald, R. L. 1966. "Lunar and Seasonal Variations in Obstetrical Factors." *J. Genet. Psychol.*, 108: 81-87.

McFarland, R. A. 1939. "The Psycho-Physiological Effects of Reduced Oxygen Pressure." *Res. Publ. Ass. Res. Nerv. Ment. Dis.*, 19: 112-143.

McKay, R. J., and J. F. Lucey. 1964. "Neonatology." *New Eng. J. Med.*, 270: 1231-1236, 1292-1298.

McKeown, Thomas, and J. R. Gibson. 1951. "Observations on All Births (23,970) in Birmingham, 1947." *British J. Prev. Soc. Med.*, 5: 98-112.

McKeown, Thomas. 1960. "Influences Affecting Pre-Natal Growth in Man," in J. M. Tanner, ed. *Human Growth*, Vol. III. New York: Pergamon Press.

McKeown, Thomas, and R. G. Record. 1953. "The Influence of Placental Size on Foetal Growth in Man, with Special Reference to Multiple Pregnancy." *J. Endocr.*, 9: 418-426.

McKeown, Thomas, and R. G. Record. 1953. "The Influence of Placental Size on Fetal Growth According to Sex and Order of Birth." *J. Endocr.*, 10: 73-81.

McLaurin, L. P., and J. R. Cotter. 1967. "Placental Transfer of Iron." *Am. J. Obstet. Gynec.*, 98: 931-937.

McLaren, Anne. 1965. "Genetic and Environmental Effects on Foetal and Placental Growth in Mice." *J. Reprod. Fert.*, 9: 79-98.

McLaren, D. S. 1959. "Records of Birth Weight and Prematurity in Wasukama of Lake Province, Tanganyika." *Trans. Roy. Soc. Trop. Med. Hyg.*, 53: 173-178.

MacMahon, Brian, Marc Alpert, and E. J. Salber. 1966. "Infant Weight and Parental Smoking Habits." *Am. J. Epidem.*, 82: 247-261.

Macedo Dianderas, Julio. 1957. "La Tension Arterial en el Nino de la Altura." *Rev. Asoc. Med. Yauli* II: 232-239.

Macedo Dianderas, Julio. 1966. "Peso, Talla, Pulso, y Presion Arterial del Recien Nacido en las Grandes Alturas." *Arch. Inst. Biol. Andina*, I: 234-237.

Makowski, E. L., F. C. Battaglia, Giacomo Meschia, R. E. Behrman, John Schruefer, A. E. Seeds, and P. D. Bruns. 1968. "Effect of Maternal Exposure to High Altitude upon Fetal Oxygenation." *Am. J. Obstet. Gynec.*, 100: 852-861.

Malpas, Percy. 1964. "Length of the Human Umbilical Cord at Term." *Brit. Med. J.*, 1: 673-674.

Malpas, Percy, and E. M. Symonds. 1966. "Observations on the

Structure of the Human Umbilical Cord." *Surg. Gynec. Obstet.*, 123: 746-750.

Marcos, P. E. 1966. "Current Views on Placenta Praevia." *Acta Med. Philipp.*, 2: 151-154.

Marticorena, E., J. Severino, D. Penaloza, and K. Hellriegel. 1959. "Influencia de las Grandes Alturas en la Determinacion de la Persistencia del Canal Arterial: Observaciones Realizadas en 3500 Escolares de Altura a 4330 Metros Sobre el Nivel del Mar." *Rev. Asoc. Med. Prov. Yauli*, IV: 37-45.

Mazess, R. B. 1966. "Neonatal Mortality and Altitude in Peru." *Am. J. Phys. Anthrop.*, 23: 209-214.

Mazess, R. B., and P. T. Baker. 1964. "Diet of Quechua Indians at High Altitude: Nunoa, Peru." *Am. J. Clin. Nutr.*, 15: 341-351.

Meredith, H. V. 1952. "North American Negro Infants: Size at Birth and Growth During the First Postnatal Year." *Hum. Biol.*, 24: 290-308.

Metcalfe, James, Giacomo Meschia, Andre Hellegers, Harry Prystowsky, William Huckabee, and D. H. Barron. 1962. "Observations on the Placental Exchange of the Respiratory Gases in Pregnant Ewes at High Altitude." *Quart. J. Exp. Physiol.*, 47: 74-92.

Metcalfe, James, M. J. Novy, and E. N. Peterson. 1967. "Reproduction at High Altitudes," in Kurt Benirschke, ed. *Comparative Aspects of Reproductive Failure.* New York: Springer-Verlag.

Miller, J. A., and Faith Miller. 1966. "Interactions Between Hypothermia and Hypoxia-Hypercapnia in Neonates." *Fed. Proc.*, 25: 1338-1341.

Millis, Jean. 1952. "A Study of the Effect of Nutrition on Fertility and the Outcome of Pregnancy in Singapore in 1947 and 1950." *Med. J. Malaya*, 6: 157-183.

Millis, Jean. 1957. "The Effect of Equatorial Climate on Birth Weight and Subsequent Weight of Infants." *J. Trop. Pediat.*, 3: 105-113.

Moncloa, F., J. Donayre, L. Sobrevilla, and R. Guerra-Garcia. 1965. "Endocrine Studies at High Altitude: Adrenal Cortical Function in Sea Level Natives Exposed to High Altitudes (4300 meters) for Two Weeks." *J. Clin. End. Metab.*, 25: 1640-1642.

Moncloa, F., R. Guerra-Garcia, C. Subauste, L. A. Sobrevilla, and J. Donayre. 1966. "Endocrine Studies at High Altitude: Thyroid Function in Sea Level Natives Exposed for Two Weeks to an Altitude of 4300 Meters." *J. Clin. End. Metab.*, 26: 1237-1239.

Monge, C. M. 1948. *Acclimatization in the Andes: Historical Con-*

firmations of 'Climatic Aggression' in the Development of Andean Man.* Baltimore: Johns Hopkins Press.

Monge, C. M. 1960. *Acclimatacion en los Andes. Extractos de Investigaciones Sobre la Biologia de Altitud.* Lima: Universidad Nacional Mayor de San Marcos.

Monge, C. M., and C. C. Monge. 1966. *High Altitude Diseases Mechanism and Management.* Springfield, Illinois: Charles Thomas.

Monge, C. M., M. San Martin, J. Atkins, and J. Castanon. 1945. "Aclimatacion del Ganado Ovino en las Grandes Alturas: Fertilidad e Infertilidad Reversible Durante la Fase Adaptiva." *An. Fac. Med. Lima,* 23: 15-31.

Montagu, M., F. Ashley. 1962. *Prenatal Influences.* Springfield, Illinois: Charles Thomas.

Moore, Carl R., and Dorothy Price. 1948. "A Study at High Altitude of Reproduction, Growth, Sexual Maturity and Organ Weights." *J. Exp. Zool.,* 108: 171-216.

Morley, David, and George Knox. 1960. "The Birth Weights of Yoruba Babies." *J. Obstet. Gynaec. Brit. Emp.,* 67: 975-979.

Morton, N. E. 1955. "The Inheritance of Human Birth Weight." *Ann. Hum. Genet.,* 20: 125-134.

Morton, N. E. 1958. "Empirical Risks in Consanguineous Marriages: Birth Weight, Gestation Time and Measurements of Infants." *Am. J. Hum. Genet.,* 10: 344-349.

Mosso, Angelo. 1898. *Life of Man in the High Alps.* Translated from the second edition of the Italian by E. Lough Kiesow. London: T. Fisher Unwin.

Naeye, R. L. 1965. "Children at High Altitude: Pulmonary and Renal Abnormalities" *Circ. Res.,* 16: 33-38.

Naeye, R. L. 1965. "Malnutrition: Probable Cause of Fetal Growth Retardation." *Arch. Path.,* 79: 284-291.

Naeye, R. L. 1966. "Abnormalities in Infants of Mothers with Toxemia of Pregnancy." *Am. J. Obstet. Gynec.,* 95: 276-283.

Naeye, R. L. 1967. "Infants of Prolonged Gestation: A Necropsy Study." *Arch. Path.,* 84: 37-41.

Nelson, Dorothy, and M. W. Burrill. 1944. "Repeated Exposures to Simulated High Altitude: Estrus Cycles and Fertility of the White Rat." *Fed. Proc.,* 3: 34-35.

Nesbitt, R. E. L., Jr. 1966. "Perinatal Development," in Frank Falkner, ed. *Human Development.* Philadelphia: W. B. Saunders.

Newsom, B. D., and D. J. Kimeldorf. 1960. "Species Differences in Altitude Tolerance Following X-Irradiation." *Am. J. Physiol.,* 198: 762-764.

Noriega Pinillos, Luis. 1961. "Aporte al Estudio del Trabajo de Parto y el Recien Nacido en la Altura." Thesis 5191, Facultad de Medicina, Lima.

North, A. F. 1966. "Small-for-Dates Neonates: Maternal, Gestational, and Neonatal Characteristics." *Pediat.,* 38: 1013-1019.

Northrup, D. W., and E. J. Van Liere. 1960. "Cardiac Hypertrophy Due to Hypoxia in Male and Female Rats." *Fed. Proc.,* 19: 111.

Oficina de Planificacion. 1965. "Nacimientos, Defunciones y Defunciones Fetales en Distritos con Certificacion Profesional." Lima: Division de Estadisticas de Salud.

Opitz, E., and Max Schneider. 1950. "The Oxygen Supply of the Brain and the Mechanism of Deficiency Effects." *Ergebn. Physiol.,* 46: 126-260.

O'Sullivan, J. B., Sydney Gellis, B. O. Tenney, and C. M. Mahon. 1965. "Aspects of Birth Weight and Its Influencing Variables." *Am. J. Obstet. Gynec.,* 92: 1023-1029.

O'Sullivan, J. B., Sydney Gellis, B. O Tenney, and C. M. Mahon. 1966. "Gestational Blood Glucose Levels in Normal and Potentially Diabetic Women Related to the Birth Weight of their Infants." *Diabetes,* 15: 466-470.

Ounsted, Margaret. 1966. "Unconstrained Foetal Growth in Man: A Preliminary Note." *Develop. Med. Child Neurol.,* 8: 3-8.

Ounsted, Margaret, and Christopher Ounsted. 1966. "Maternal Regulation of Intra-Uterine Growth." *Nature,* 212: 995-997.

Page, E. W. 1967. "Autonomic Innervation of the Human Placenta," in R. M. Wynn, ed. *Fetal Homeostasis,* Vol. Two. New York: New York Academy of Sciences Interdisciplinary Communications Program.

Patten, B. M. 1953. *Human Embryology.* New York: McGraw-Hill.

Penrose, L. S. 1951. "Data on the Genetics of Birth Weight." *Ann. Eugenics,* 16: 378-381.

Penrose, L. S. 1961. "Genetics of Growth and Development of the Foetus," in L. S. Penrose, ed. *Recent Advances in Human Genetics.* Boston: Little, Brown and Company.

Perrin, E. B., and M. C. Sheps. 1965. "A Mathematical Model for Human Fertility Patterns." *Arch. Environ. Health,* 10: 694-698.

Platt, B. S. 1966. "Congenital Protein-Calorie Deficiency." *Proc. Roy. Soc. Med.,* 59: 1077-1079.

Potter, E. L. 1961. *Pathology of the Fetus and Infant*. Chicago: Year Book Publishers.

Price, Richard. 1965. "Trial Marriage in the Andes." *Ethnology*, IV: 310-322.

Ramaiah, T. J., and V. L. Narsimham. 1967. "Birth Weight as a Measure of Prematurity and Its Relationship with Certain Maternal Factors." *Ind. J. Med. Res.*, 55: 513-524.

Ravenholt, R. T., Mary J. Levinski, D. J. Nellist, and Maxine Takenaga. 1966. "Effects of Smoking upon Reproduction." *Am. J. Obstet. Gynec.*, 96: 267-281.

Reed, T. E. 1967. "Research on Blood Groups and Selection from the Child Health and Development Studies, Oakland, California. Infant Birth Measurements." *Am. J. Hum. Genet.*, 19: 732-746.

Reynafarge, Cesar. 1959. "Bone-Marrow Studies in the Newborn Infant at High Altitudes." *J. Pediat.*, 54: 152-161.

Richardson, S. A., and A. F. Guttmacher, eds. 1967. *Childbearing —Its Social and Psychological Aspects*. New York: The Williams and Wilkins Company.

Roberts, D. F., and Tanner, R. E. 1963. "Effects of Parity on Birth Weight and Other Variables in a Tanganyika Bantu Sample." *Brit. J. Prev. Soc. Med.*, 17: 209-215.

Roberts, J. C., R. J. Hock, and R. E. Smith. 1966. "Seasonal Metabolic Responses of Deer Mice (Peromyscus) to Temperature and Altitude." *Fed. Proc.*, 25: 1275-1286.

Robinson, Derek. 1967. "Precedents of Fetal Death." *Am. J. Obstet. Gynec.*, 97: 936-942.

Robson, E. B. 1955. "Birth Weight in Cousins." *Ann. Hum. Gen.*, 19: 262-268.

Rosa, Franz, and Leah Resnick. 1965. "Birth Weight and Perinatal Mortality in the American Indian." *Am. J. Obstet. Gynec.*, 91: 972-976.

Rosen, Marvin, E. F. Downs, F .D. Napolitani, and D. P. Swartz. 1968. "The Quality of Reproduction in an Urban Indigent Population: Birth Weight: The Differences Between Mothers of Low-Weight and of Term-Size Infants." *Obstet. Gynec.*, 31: 276-282.

Salber, E. J., and E. S. Bradshaw. 1951. "Birth Weights of South African Babies." *Brit. J. Prev. Soc. Med*, 5: 113-119.

Sanchez Kong, R. A. 1963. "Estudio Macroscopico de 100 Placentas en la Hospital 'Esperanza' de Cerro de Pasco." Thesis 5608, Facultad de Medicina, Lima.

Sarram, Mahmood, and Mohammed Saadatnejadi. 1967. "Birth

Weight in Shiraz (Iran) in Relation to Maternal Socioeconomic Status." *Obstet. Gynec.*, 30: 367-370.

Schaffer, Karl E., ed. 1962. *Environmental Effects on Consciousness.* New York: The MacMillan Company.

Schneider, Jan. 1968. "Low Birth Weight Infants." *Obstet. Gynec.*, 31: 283-287.

Schultz, A. H. 1926. "Fetal Growth of Man and Other Primates." *Quart. Rev. Biol.*, 1: 465-521.

Sehgal, A. K., Iqbal Krishan, R. P. Malhotra, and H. D. Gupta. 1968. "Observations on the Blood Pressure of Tibetans." *Circulation*, 37: 36-44.

Seller, M. J., and R. G. Spector. 1964. "The Effects of Anoxia on the Newborn and Adult Rat Lung." *J. Path. Bact.*, 88: 309-311.

Sinclair, J. G. 1948. "Placental-Fetal Weight Ratios." *Texas Rep. Biol. Med.*, 6: 168-175.

Sinclair, J. G. 1948. "Significance of Placental and Birth Weight Ratios." *Anat. Rec.*, 102: 245-258.

Smith, A. H., and U. K. Abbott. 1961. "Adaptation of the Domestic Fowl to High Altitude." *Poultry Sci.*, 40: 1459.

Sobrevilla, L. A., I. Romero, F. Moncloa, J. Donayre, and R. Guerra-Garcia. 1967. "Endocrine Studies at High Altitude. Urinary Gonadotrophins in Subjects Native to and Living at 14,000 Feet and During Acute Exposure of Men Living at Sea Level to High Altitudes." *Acta Endocr.*, 56: 369-375.

Spencer, R. P. 1968. "Placental Growth: Semiquantitative Approaches." *Biol. Neonat.*, 12: 180-185.

Standard, K. L., V. G. Wills, and J. C. Waterlow. 1959. "Indirect Indicators of Muscle Mass in Malnourished Infants." *Am. J. Clin. Nutr.*, 7: 271-279.

Stickney, J. C., T. L. Browne, and E. J. Van Liere. 1962. "The Effect of Intermittent Exposures to Simulated High Altitude upon Lactation in the Goat." *Proc. W. Va. Acad. Sci.*, 34: 7-12.

Stickney, J. C., T. L Browne, and E. J. Van Liere. 1962. "Erythropoietin in Goats at Simulated High Altitude," in W. H. Weihe, ed. *The Physiological Effects of High Altitude.* New York: Pergamon Press.

Stycos, J. Mayone. 1968. *Human Fertility in Latin America: Sociological Perspectives.* Ithaca, New York: Cornell University Press.

Taff, M. A., Jr., and C. L. Wilbar, Jr. 1953. "Immaturity of Single Live Births According to Weight, with Particular Reference to Race." *Am. J. Dis. Child,* 85: 279-284.

Tanner, J. M. 1960. "Genetics of Human Growth," in J. M. Tanner, ed. *Human Growth,* Vol. III. New York: Pergamon Press.

Tanner, J. M. 1966. "Growth and Physique in Different Populations of Mankind," in P. T. Baker and J. S. Weiner, eds. *The Biology of Human Adaptability.* Oxford: Clarendon Press.

Tenney, S. M., and J. E. Remmers. 1966. "Alveolar Dimensions in the Lungs of Animals Raised at High Altitudes." *J. Appl. Physiol.,* 21: 1328-1330.

Theobald, G. W. 1965. "Reproductive Ability in Woman." *Am. J. Obstet. Gynec.,* 92: 332-340.

Thompson, Barbara, and Sir Dugald Baird. 1967. "Some Impressions on Childbearing in Tropical Areas: I. Description of Populations and Data Available. II. Pre-Eclampsia and Low Birth Weight. III. Outcome of Labor." *J. Obstet. Gynaec. Brit. Comm.,* 74: 329-338, 499-509, 510-522.

Thomson, A. M., Daphne Chun, and Sir Dugald Baird. 1963. "Perinatal Mortality in Hong Kong and in Aberdeen, Scotland." *J. Obstet. Gynaec. Brit. Comm.,* 70: 871-877.

Timiras, P. S. 1962. "Comparison of Growth and Development of the Rat at High Altitude and at Sea Level," in W. H. Weihe, ed. *The Physiological Effects of High Altitude.* New York: Pergamon Press.

Timiras, P. S., and D. E. Woolley. 1966. "Functional and Morphologic Development of Brain and Other Organs of Rats at High Altitude." *Fed. Proc.,* 25: 1312-1320.

Tominaga, Toshiro, and E. W. Page. 1966. "Accommodation of the Human Placenta to Hypoxia." *Am. J. Obstet. Gynec.,* 94: 679-691.

Torpin, Richard, and Bruce Swain. 1966. "Placental Infarction in 1,000 Cases Correlated with the Clinical Findings." *Am. J. Obstet. Gynec.,* 94: 284-285.

Treloar, A. E., B. G. Behn, and D. W. Cowan. 1967. "Analysis of Gestational Interval." *Am. J. Obstet. Gynec,.* 99: 34-45.

Tremblay, P. C., Stella Sylewsky, and G. B. Maughan. 1965. "Role of the Placenta in Fetal Malnutrition." *Am. J. Obstet. Gynec.,* 91: 597-605.

Tschopik, Harry, Jr. 1947. "The Aymara," in Julian H. Steward, ed. *Handbook of South American Indians.* Bureau of American Ethnology Bull. 143, Vol. 2, Washington, D. C.

Usher, Robert, Frances McLean, and K. E. Scott. 1966. "Judgment of Fetal Age. Clinical Significance of Gestational Age and an

Objective Method for Its Assessment." *Pediat. Clin. N. Amer.,* 13: 835-848.

United States Department of Health, Education, and Welfare. 1965. "Weight at Birth and Survival of the Newborn." Public Health Service Publication 1000, Series 21, No. 3, Washington, D. C.

Valsik, J. A. 1965. "The Seasonal Rhythm of Menarche: A Review." *Hum. Biol.,* 37: 75-90.

Van Den Berg, B. J., and J. Yerushalmy. 1966. "The Relationship of the Rate of Intrauterine Growth of Infants of Low Birth Weight to Mortality, Morbidity, and Congenital Anomalies." *J. Pediat.,* 69: 531-545.

Van Liere, E. J., and J. C. Stickney, 1963. *Hypoxia.* Chicago: University of Chicago Press.

Vilchez, Horacio. 1961. "Caracteres Fisicos de la Placenta y el Cordon en Nuestro Medio." Thesis 2702, Facultad de Medicina, Lima.

Villee, C. A. 1960. *The Placenta and Fetal Membranes.* New York: Williams and Wilkins Company.

Vincent, M., and J. Ghesquiere. 1962. "The Newborn Pigmy and His Mother." *Am J. Phys. Anthrop.,* 20: 237-247.

Walker, C. W., and B. G. Pye, 1960. "The Length of the Human Umbilical Cord: A Statistical Report." *Brit. Med. J.,* 1: 546-548.

Walker, James. "The 'Small for Dates' Baby." *Proc. Roy. Soc. Med.,* 60: 877-879.

Walker, James, and A. C. Turnbull, eds. 1959. *Oxygen Supply to the Human Foetus.* Oxford: Blackwell.

Warkany, Josef, B. B. Monroe, and B. S. Sutherland. 1961. "Intra-Uterine Growth Retardation." *Am. J. Dis. Child.,* 102: 249-279.

Weihe, W. H. 1962. "Some Examples of Endocrine and Metabolic Functions in Rats During Acclimatization to High Altitude," in W. H. Weihe, ed. *The Physiological Effects of High Altitude.* New York: Pergamon Press.

Weiner, J. S. 1964. "Human Ecology," in G. A. Harrison, J. S. Weiner, J. M. Tanner, and N. A. Barnicot, eds. *Human Biology.* New York: Oxford University Press.

Widdowson, E. M., and R. A. McCance. 1960. "Some Effects of Accelerating Growth. General Somatic Development." *Proc. Roy. Soc. Biol.,* 152: 188-206.

Wigglesworth, J. S. 1964. "Morphological Variations in the Insufficient Placenta." *J. Obstet. Gynaec. Brit. Comm.,* 71: 871-884.

Wigglesworth, J. S. 1967. "Pathological and Experimental Aspects of Foetal Growth Retardation." *Proc. Roy. Soc. Med.*, 60: 879-881.

Wislocki, G. B. 1929. "On the Placentation of Primates, with a Consideration of the Phylogeny of the Placenta." *Carnegie Cont. Emb.*, 20: 51-80.

Wolstenholme, G. E. W., and Maeve O'Connor, eds. 1965. *Ciba Foundation Symposium on Preimplantation Stages of Pregnancy.* Boston: Little, Brown and Company.

World Health Organization. 1960. *Endemic Goitre.* Geneva: World Health Organization.

World Health Organization. 1961. "Public Health Aspects of Low Birth Weight: Third Report of the Expert Committee on Maternal and Child Health." *WHO Tech. Rep.*, 217: 1-16.

Yerushalmy, J. 1967. "The Classification of Newborn Infants by Birth Weight and Gestational Age." *J. Pediat.*, 71: 164-172.

Index

141

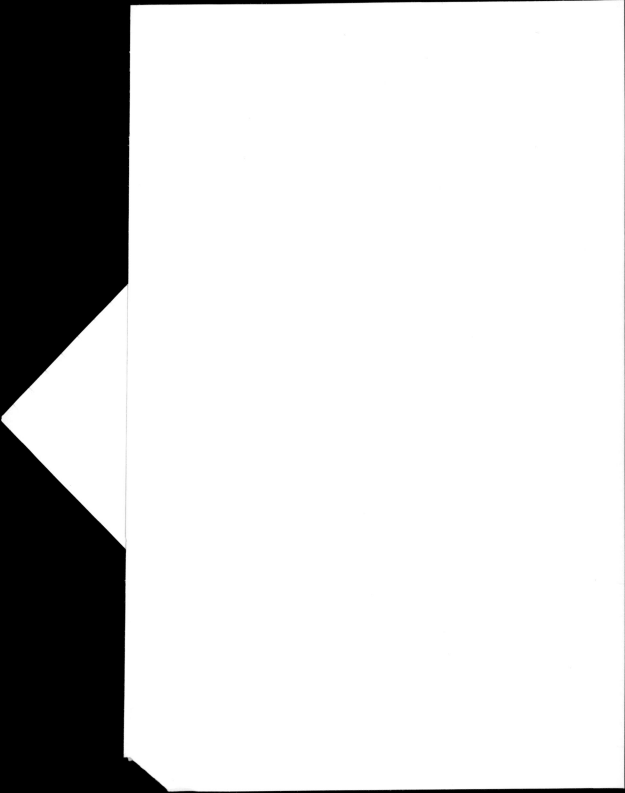

Date D

DE 22 '72 12/13